Melanoma

Melanoma

Jonathan S. Zager

Ragini R. Kudchadkar

Vernon K. Sondak

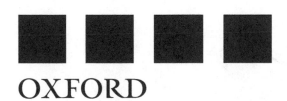

OXFORD

UNIVERSITY PRESS

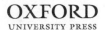

OXFORD
UNIVERSITY PRESS

Oxford University Press is a department of the University of Oxford. It furthers
the University's objective of excellence in research, scholarship, and education
by publishing worldwide.Oxford is a registered trade mark of Oxford University
Press in the UK and certain other countries.

Published in the United States of America by Oxford University Press
198 Madison Avenue, New York, NY 10016, United States of America.

© Oxford University Press 2016

First Edition published in 2016

Library of Congress Cataloging-in-Publication Data
Melanoma (Sondak)
Melanoma/[edited by] Jonathan S. Zager, Ragini R. Kudchadkar, Vernon K.
Sondak.
  p. ; cm.
Includes bibliographical references.
ISBN 978-0-19-997101-5
I. Zager, Jonathan S., editor.   II. Kudchadkar, Ragini, editor.   III. Sondak,
Vernon K., 1957–, editor.   IV. Title.
[DNLM: 1. Melanoma—therapy.   2. Melanoma—diagnosis.   QZ 200]
RC280.M37
616.99'477—dc23
2015009687

9 8 7 6 5 4 3 2 1

Printed by Sheridan, USA

Contents

Principal Editors

Jonathan S. Zager, MD, FACS

Chair of Graduate Medical Education
Director of Regional Therapies
Senior Member
Department of Cutaneous Oncology
Moffitt Cancer Center
Professor of Surgery
University of South Florida, Morsani College of Medicine
Tampa, Florida

Ragini R. Kudchadkar, MD

Assistant Professor of Hematology/Oncology
Winship Cancer Institute
Emory University
Atlanta, Georgia

Vernon K. Sondak, MD

Chair, Department of Cutaneous Oncology
Director of Surgical Education
H. Lee Moffitt Cancer Center
Professor, Department of Surgery and Oncologic Sciences
University of South Florida, Morsani College of Medicine
Tampa, Florida

Contributors

Alia Abdulla, DO

Medical Director of Surgical
    Oncology
North Shore Medical Center
Department of Surgical Oncology
Center for Advanced Surgical
    Oncology
Palmetto General Hospital
Hialeah, Florida

Michelle Ashworth, MD

Clinical Fellow
Hematology & Oncology Fellow
University of California
San Francisco, California

Kathryn Baksh, MD

Hematology/Oncology Staff
    Physician
Department of Hematology and
    Medical Oncology
James A. Haley Veterans
    Administration
University of South Florida
Tampa, Florida

Richard D. Carvajal, MD

Director, Melanoma and
    Experimental Therapeutics
    Services
Assistant Professor of Medicine
Columbia University Medical Center
New York, New York

Michael D. Chuong, MD

Department of Radiation Oncology
University of Maryland
    Medical Center
Baltimore, Maryland

Adil Daud, MD

Director, Melanoma Clinical
    Research
UCSF Helen Diller Family
    Comprehensive Cancer Center
San Francisco, California

Maggie Diller, MD

Cutaneous Oncology Fellow
Department of Surgical Oncology
Winship Cancer Institute
Emory University
Atlanta, Georgia

Matthew P. Doepker, MD

Cutaneous Oncology Program
H. Lee Moffitt Cancer Center
Tampa, Florida

Jeffrey M. Farma, MD

Department of Surgical Oncology
Associate Professor
Fox Chase Cancer Center
Philadelphia, Pennsylvania

Peter A. Forsyth, MD

Department of Neuro-Oncology
H. Lee Moffitt Cancer Center
Oncologic Sciences
University of South Florida College
    of Medicine
Tampa, Florida

Emmanuel Gabriel, MD, PhD

Fellow in Complex Surgical
    Oncology
Department of Surgical Oncology
Roswell Park Cancer Institute
Buffalo, New York

Nicole Howe, MD
Procedural Dermatology Fellow
The University of Vermont
    Medical Center
Burlington, Vermont

Mohammad K. Khan, MD, PhD, DABR
Department of Radiation Oncology
Assistant Professor and Medical
    Student Clerkship Director
Winship Cancer Institute
Emory University School of
    Medicine
Atlanta, Georgia

Timothy McCardle, MD
Department of Pathology
H. Lee Moffitt Cancer Center
Tampa, Florida

Fariba Navid, MD
Associate Member
Department of Oncology
St. Jude Children's Research
    Hospital
Memphis, Tennessee

Prejesh Philips, MD
Assistant Professor of Surgery
Division of Surgical Oncology
Department of Surgery
University of Louisville School of
    Medicine
Louisville, Kentucky

Carlos Prieto-Granada, MD
Dermatopathology Fellow
Department of Pathology
Moffitt Cancer Center
University of South Florida
Tampa, Florida

Nikhil G. Rao, MD
Department of Radiation Oncology
H. Lee Moffitt Cancer Center
Tampa, Florida

Damon Reed, MD
Director of the Adolescent and
    Young Adult Program
Sarcoma Department and
    Cutaneous Oncology
H. Lee Moffitt Cancer Center and
    Research Institute
Tampa, Florida

Solmaz Sahebjam, MD
Department of Neuro-Oncology
H. Lee Moffitt Cancer Center
Oncologic Sciences
University of South Florida College
    of Medicine
Tampa, Florida

Alfredo A. Santillan, MD, MPH
Associate Professor of Surgery
Department of Surgical Oncology
    and Endocrine Surgery
University of Texas Health Science
    Center
San Antonio, Texas

Amod A. Sarnaik, MD
Cutaneous Oncology Program
H. Lee Moffitt Cancer Center
Tampa, Florida

Alexander N. Shoushtari, MD
Assistant Attending Physician
Melanoma and Immunotherapeutics
    Service
Memorial Sloan Kettering
    Cancer Center
New York, New York
Weill Cornell Medical College
New York, New York

Maki Yamamoto, MD
Health Sciences Clinical Assistant
    Professor
Associate Program Director
Associate Director of the
    Melanoma Center
UC Irvine Health
University of California, Irvine

x

Chapter 1

Epidemiology, Risk Factors, and Clinical Presentation of Melanoma

Maki Yamamoto and Vernon K. Sondak

Epidemiology

There were a projected 76,100 new cases of invasive cutaneous melanoma in the United States in 2014, with an additional 63,770 cases of newly diagnosed melanoma in situ.[1] Excluding basal and squamous cell carcinomas, this becomes the fifth and seventh most common malignancy in males and females, respectively. Unlike the declining rates in most other cancer types (such as prostate, colorectal, lung), the incidence of melanoma has been increasing, with an estimated annual percentage change ranging from 1.7–2.4%. Based on the National Cancer Institute's (NCI) Surveillance, Epidemiology, and End Results (SEER) data collected from 2008 to 2010, males have a 2.9% (1 in 34) lifetime risk of developing melanoma, while females have a slightly lower lifetime risk of 1.9% (1 in 53).[1] Compared to the more common basal and squamous cell carcinomas, melanoma accounts for only about 3% of all skin cancers. Despite the lower incidence of all skin cancers, melanoma accounts for the majority of cancer-related deaths.[2]

The age of peak incidence of melanoma is 55–64 years, with a median age of diagnosis at 61.[3] Prognosis is related to the patient's age at the time of melanoma diagnosis. A recent study by Balch et al.[4] evaluated 11,088 melanoma patients according to their age, grouped by decades. The authors showed that elderly patients (>70 years of age) had a propensity for melanomas with more aggressive pathological features and with an associated poorer survival rate. Teenagers and younger children have melanomas with a worse stage at presentation of disease[5] but, paradoxically, have a more favorable survival outcome than their more elderly counterparts.[4,5] Whether due to coexisting medical conditions, different tumor biology, or waning immune competency, the reasons for this poorer prognosis in elderly patients is unclear.

Gender differences exist in melanoma incidence as well. The lifetime probability for developing melanoma is higher in males than in females: 2.9 vs. 1.9%.[1] The higher incidence in males also translates to a higher mortality rate. The number of deaths per 100,000 persons was 4.1 in males, but only 1.7 in females.[3] The greater mortality rate cannot be explained by incidence alone. Multiple studies have evaluated various tumor- and patient-related factors (Breslow thickness, ulceration, mitotic rate, histological subtype, age, and gender) on long-term prognosis.[6] Male gender has been shown multiple times to have a worse prognosis compared to females'.[7] A study evaluating 3,324 patients showed worse disease-free survival and overall survival rates in males ($P < 0.001$) after adjusting for other prognostic factors.[8]

Racial disparities also exist in the incidence and prognosis for patients with cutaneous melanoma.[9] Primary cutaneous melanoma is predominantly encountered in white patients. A 10-year SEER database study illustrated the differences: age-adjusted melanoma incidence per 100,000 persons was 18.4 for whites, while that for Hispanics and African Americans were considerably less, at 2.3 and 0.8, respectively.[10] In addition, the presentation of disease differs within ethnic groups in regard to primary tumor location, histological subtype, and stage of disease. While the trunk is the most common location for the primary tumor in white patients, Hispanics and African Americans have a greater propensity to lesions on their lower extremities.[10,11] Although acral lentiginous melanoma (ALM) is the least common of the four major histological subtypes, the proportion of ALM cases is highest in ethnic minorities; with African Americans composing 36% of all ALM cases, according to recent SEER data.[12] More importantly, inequities in stage at time of presentation and in survival rates by stage exist for minority groups. Minority patients have significantly higher odds for presenting with distant metastases than do white patients (odds ratios of 3.6 and 4.2 for Hispanics and African Americans, respectively).[10] Although there is a higher risk for later stage of presentation with minority groups, even adjusting for age, sex, anatomical site, histological subtype, stage of disease, and socioeconomic status, African Americans still had a significantly increased risk of death.[10,13] Due to the relative rarity of melanoma in minority groups, it is unclear to what degree tumor biology, socioeconomic status, availability of treatment options, and later stage of presentation are each responsible for the poorer survival of patients in certain ethnic groups.

Risk Factors

Although considerable research is ongoing as to the prevention and tumorigenesis of melanoma, several environmental, genetic, and other risk factors are well documented. By identifying groups of patients at high risk, targeted screening practices could potentially lead to earlier diagnosis of melanoma.

Melanoma has long been associated with ultraviolet (UV) exposure. The wavelengths of ultraviolet radiation range from 100–400 nm. They are further classified according to wavelength, into UV-A (320–400 nm), UV-B (290–320 nm), and UV-C (100–290 nm). The ozone layer filters out virtually all the UV-C and the majority of the UV-B radiation reaching the Earth's surface; the remaining fraction of UV-B and all of the UV-A radiation have been implicated in the development of cutaneous malignancies, including cutaneous melanoma.[14] Although only a small percentage of UV-B radiation reaches the Earth's surface, it is considered the major contributor to melanoma risk due to induction of DNA damage. To a lesser degree, melanoma development also is attributable to UV-A radiation exposure by its production of free radicals and immunosuppressive effects. A variety of animal studies have shown the development of melanoma with exposure to UV-B and UV-A radiation.[15,16] The amount of UV radiation exposure correlates with the increased risk for melanoma development.[17] Studies evaluating closer proximity to the equator and higher altitude areas show an increased incidence of melanoma in these areas.[18]

UV exposure is not solely due to natural sources, especially with the increasing popularity of indoor tanning. Nearly 30 million people utilize indoor tanning salons in the United States each year; 2.3 million of these are adolescents.[19] Similar to solar sources, modern tanning equipment emits predominantly in the UV-A range, with a small percentage in the UV-B. However, the intensity of the UV radiation from sunbeds or tanning beds (especially in the UV-A spectrum) can be 10–15 times higher than normal midday sun exposure.[20] A recent meta-analysis evaluating 27 international studies showed an increased relative risk of 1.20 (95% confidence interval 1.08–1.34) with any use of sunbeds for the development of melanoma.[21] The risk was dose-dependent; it increased by 1.8% for each additional sunbed session per year. The exposure to sunbeds was even more crucial in the young: relative risk increased to 1.87 with first-ever use of sunbeds prior to the age of 35. Some confounding factors may be that patients with certain phenotypical characteristics such as fair skin, red or blonde hair, and increased freckling are more apt to practice indoor tanning.[22] In addition, use of sunbeds may be a marker for increased sun exposure as a part of an unhealthy lifestyle.[23]

The presence of dysplastic nevi confers an increased risk in the development of melanoma; the risk increases linearly with the number of nevi present.[24] Some have theorized that dysplastic nevi lie on a spectrum between common nevi and melanoma.[25] However, the overwhelming majority of dysplastic nevi do not transform into melanoma. In addition, there remains debate as to the proper nomenclature for dysplastic nevi and their associated syndromes, such as atypical mole (and syndrome), Clark nevus, dysplastic nevi (and syndrome), B-K mole syndrome, and more recently, familial atypical multiple mole and melanoma syndrome (FAMM). First described in 1820 by Norris[26] and further characterized by Clark[27] and Lynch,[28] FAMM was described as the presence of melanoma in first-degree relatives, a large number of melanocytic nevi (>50), and architectural disorder and atypia. Although the exact genes responsible for melanoma development have not been elucidated, one candidate gene identified through analysis of pedigrees of FAMM is cyclin-dependent kinase inhibitor 2A (CDKN2A). CDKN2A mutations account for 20–40% of hereditary melanoma.[29]

Clinical Presentation

With the increasing incidence of melanoma in the United States, emphasis remains on early diagnosis by patients, dermatologists, and primary care physicians. Long-term survival for patients with metastatic melanoma—despite advances in treatment—is still poor, while those with early localized melanoma carry an excellent prognosis. There is clear evidence for a direct correlation between survival and tumor thickness at diagnosis. As Breslow depth increases, survival rates decline, ranging from 92% 10-year survival for T1 melanomas (≤1.00 mm) to 50% for T4 melanomas (>4 mm).[30] Nodal status of the draining lymphatic basin also shows a direct correlation to long-term survival. Micrometastatic disease is associated with a 70% five-year survival, which worsens to 39% for patients with multiple/matted nodes or in-transit disease.[30] This makes early diagnosis imperative in improving survival rates for melanoma.

Early clinical recognition of suspicious pigmented lesions with liberal usage of biopsy is essential to the early diagnosis of melanoma. Several mnemonics and tools have been developed to help the dermatologist and primary care physician recognize suspicious lesions that require biopsy for confirmation. The most well-known of these is the ABCD acronym (**A**symmetry, **B**order irregularity, **C**olor variegation, and **D**iameter), which was recently expanded to include a fifth criterion, **E** (**E**volving lesion)[31,32] (see Table 1.1). Most melanomas grow at an irregular rate, resulting in asymmetry and irregular borders that differ from those of benign lesions, which tend to be round, symmetrical, and of uniform color throughout, with smooth borders. Melanomas tend to have variable hues throughout the lesion, and usually present with diameters of at least 6 mm (see Figure 1.1). It should be emphasized that not all five criteria are found in every melanoma, and some benign lesions may possess many or all of the criteria as well. Sensitivity and specificity vary, depending on the number and combination of criteria used in the clinical evaluation for

Table 1.1 Diagnostic Algorithms for Early Detection of Cutaneous Melanoma

	Criteria
ABCDEs	A: asymmetry
	B: border irregularity
	C: color variegation
	D: diameter ≥6 mm
	E: evolving lesion
Glasgow 7-Point Checklist	Major signs:
	–Change in size
	–Change in shape
	–Change in color
	Minor signs:
	–Inflammation
	–Crusting or bleeding
	–Sensory change
	–Diameter ≥7 mm
Ugly Duckling sign	Pigmented lesion that looks different from neighboring lesions is probably malignant

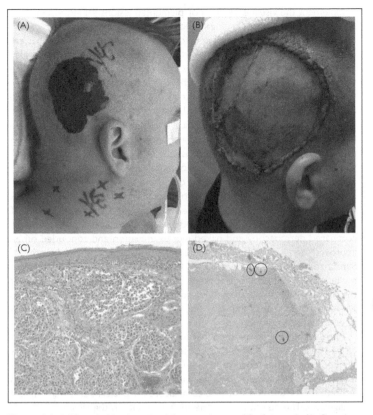

Figure 1.1 A 31-year-old male with a 4.9 mm melanoma (*C*) of the scalp (*A*, *C*), and after split thickness skin graft and sentinel node biopsy from the right neck (*B*). Three out of four sentinel nodes were positive for melanoma (*D*). Circles indicate nodal metastases shown on Melan-A stain. Images *C* and *D* courtesy of Jane Messina, MD.

suspicious lesions.[32,33] Critics of the ABCDE mnemonic have pointed out that many benign and malignant conditions, such as amelanotic melanoma, seborrheic keratosis, and atypical nevi, do not always follow the rules illustrated by the classic ABCDE of melanoma.

Other diagnostic tools have been developed for physicians to increase the early diagnosis of melanoma. Two other well-known criteria are called the Glasgow 7-Point list and the "ugly duckling" sign. The Glasgow 7-Point checklist consists of three major signs (change in size, change in shape, change in color) and four minor signs (inflammation, crusting or bleeding, sensory change, and diameter ≥7 mm).[34] The Glasgow 7-Point checklist is not widely adopted, possibly due to its greater complexity of use than the simpler ABDCE criteria.[35] The "ugly duckling" sign is based on the even simpler premise that melanoma tends to look different from the neighboring benign pigmented lesions.[36]

Recently, usage of dermoscopy (otherwise known as dermatoscopy, epiluminescence microscopy, or skin surface microscopy) has increased to complement the visual evaluation of pigmented lesions.[37] Dermoscopy is a noninvasive means of evaluating suspicious lesions by using magnification and light to visualize structures in the epidermis and superficial dermis that are not otherwise visible on routine naked-eye examinations. Traditional dermoscopes use non-polarized light sources and require an oil or alcohol interface to facilitate direct contact between the skin and the device. More recently, development of polarized light sources has eliminated the need for a liquid medium and, oftentimes, these can be attached to a digital photographic device for storage of images for medical record documentation, comparison to future physical examinations, and requests for second opinions via telemedicine consultations. Since dermoscopy evaluation by clinicians requires some degree of advanced training, computer-assisted programs have been developed to automate the analysis of dermoscopic images of pigmented lesions—with variable results.[38,39] Proponents of dermoscopy believe that it aids in the earlier detection of melanoma while decreasing biopsies of benign lesions.[37,40] Several randomized clinical trials and meta-analyses have compared dermoscopy and naked-eye examination and concluded on an improved sensitivity and specificity utilizing dermoscopy in physical exam.[41–43] Similar to algorithms and mnemonics for naked-eye examinations, there are multiple systems used in dermoscopy based on the training and education of the primary care physician and dermatologist.[37] Caution must be exercised with those melanomas that may not exhibit the typical malignant features (e.g., amelanotic melanoma).

More recently, a computer-aided multispectral skin lesion analysis device called Melafind (MELA Sciences, Inc., Irvington, New York) was approved by the Food and Drug Administration (FDA). It uses light at 10 different wavelengths, from blue (430 nm) to near-infrared (950 nm), to penetrate up to 2.5 mm below the skin's surface to evaluate for patterns that may suggest malignancy. The device assigns one of two results to the clinician: (1) consider biopsy (positive), versus (2) consider close follow-up (negative).[44,45] In a recent study by Monheit et al., a prospective, blinded, multicenter study evaluated 1,831 pigmented lesions in 1,383 patients, comparing Melafind's results to a smaller, randomly selected subset of images and patient information for dermatologists' opinions.[46] The study found a superior biopsy sensitivity and specificity for Melafind compared to clinicians viewing images of atypical pigmented lesions. A criticism of the study, however, notes that only lesions scheduled for biopsy were used for the trial. Therefore, the lesions were atypical enough to warrant biopsy and were possibly not representative of the general population. Currently, Melafind is not reimbursed by all insurance providers, and cost to the patient may limit its usage.

Conclusion

The incidence of melanoma has been slowly increasing in the United States. Melanoma can affect all age groups, including children. Poor prognostic factors include male gender, older age, increased Breslow thickness, ulceration of primary tumor, and nodal metastases. Identifying patients who are at higher risk for developing melanoma may help identify the population requiring closer screening programs. Patients with excessive ultraviolet radiation exposure (solar or artificial), dysplastic nevi, or a personal or family history of melanoma are at an increased risk for developing melanoma. Various diagnostic tools can aid the clinical examination for primary care physicians and dermatologists, such as the ABCDEs, the Glasgow 7-Point checklist, and the ugly duckling sign. Dermoscopy is being increasingly used to complement the naked-eye physical examination for the diagnosis of melanoma. Computer-assisted analysis of dermoscopic images and multispectral skin lesion analysis can be useful adjuncts but should not replace clinical examinations by experienced dermatologists.

References

1. Siegel R Ma J, Zou Z, et al. Cancer statistics, 2014. *CA Cancer J Clin*. 2014;64(1):9–29.

2. Cummins DL, Cummins JM, Pantle H, et al. Cutaneous malignant melanoma. *Mayo Clin Proc*. 2006;81(4):500–507.

3. Melanoma of the Skin: SEER Stat Fact Sheets. [February 24, 2014]; Available from: seer.cancer.gov/statfacts/html/melan.html.

4. Balch CM, Soong SJ, Gershenwald JE, et al. Age as a prognostic factor in patients with localized melanoma and regional metastases. *Ann Surg Oncol*. 2013;20(12):3961–3968.

5. Balch CM, Thompson JF, Gershenwald JE, et al. Age as a predictor of sentinel node metastasis among patients with localized melanoma: an inverse correlation of melanoma mortality and incidence of sentinel node metastasis among young and old patients. *Ann Surg Oncol*. 2014;21(4):1075–1081.

6. Gershenwald JE, Thompson W, Mansfield PF, et al. Multi-institutional melanoma lymphatic mapping experience: the prognostic value of sentinel lymph node status in 612 stage I or II melanoma patients. *J Clin Oncol*. 1999;17(3):976–983.

7. Balch CM, Buzaid AC, Soong SJ, et al. Final version of the American Joint Committee on Cancer staging system for cutaneous melanoma. *J Clin Oncol*. 2001;19(16):3635–3648.

8. Scoggins CR, Ross MI, Reintgen DS, et al. Gender-related differences in outcome for melanoma patients. *Ann Surg*. 2006;243(5):693–98; discussion, 698–700.

9. Shoo BA, Kashani-Sabet M. Melanoma arising in African-, Asian-, Latino- and Native-American populations. *Semin Cutan Med Surg*. 2009;28(2):96–102.

10. Cormier JN, Xing Y, Ding M, et al. Ethnic differences among patients with cutaneous melanoma. *Arch Intern Med*. 2006;166(17):1907–1914.

11. Myles ZM, Buchanan N, King JB, et al. Anatomic distribution of malignant melanoma on the non-Hispanic black patient, 1998–2007. *Arch Dermatol*. 2012;148(7):797–801.

12. Bradford PT, Goldstein AM, McMaster ML, et al. Acral lentiginous melanoma: incidence and survival patterns in the United States, 1986–2005. *Arch Dermatol*. 2009;145(4):427–434.

13. Zell JA, Cinar P, Mobasher M, et al. Survival for patients with invasive cutaneous melanoma among ethnic groups: the effects of socioeconomic status and treatment. *J Clin Oncol*. 2008;26(1):66–75.

14. Mulliken JS, Russak JE, Rigel DS. The effect of sunscreen on melanoma risk. *Dermatol Clin*. 2012;30(3):369–376.

15. Klein-Szanto AJ, Silvers WK, Mintz B. Ultraviolet radiation-induced malignant skin melanoma in melanoma-susceptible transgenic mice. *Cancer Res*. 1994;54(17):4569–4572.

16. Setlow RB, Grist E, Thompson K, et al. Wavelengths effective in induction of malignant melanoma. *Proc Natl Acad Sci U S A*. 1993;90(14):6666–6670.

17. Russak JE, Rigel DS. Risk factors for the development of primary cutaneous melanoma. *Dermatol Clin*. 2012;30(3):363–368.

18. Rigel DS, Rigel EG, Rigel AC. Effects of altitude and latitude on ambient UVB radiation. *J Am Acad Dermatol*. 1999;40(1):114–116.

19. Levine JA, Sorace M, Spencer J, et al. The indoor UV tanning industry: a review of skin cancer risk, health benefit claims, and regulation. *J Am Acad Dermatol*. 2005;53(6):1038–1044.

20. Gerber B, Mathys P, Moser M, et al. Ultraviolet emission spectra of sunbeds. *Photochem Photobiol*. 2002;76(6):664–668.

21. Boniol M, Autier P, Boyle P, et al. Cutaneous melanoma attributable to sunbed use: systematic review and meta-analysis. *BMJ*. 2012;345:e4757.

22. Ezzedine K, Malvy D, Mauger E, et al. Artificial and natural ultraviolet radiation exposure: beliefs and behaviour of 7200 French adults. *J Eur Acad Dermatol Venereol*. 2008;22(2):186–194.

23. Schneider S, Kramer H. Who uses sunbeds? A systematic literature review of risk groups in developed countries. *J Eur Acad Dermatol Venereol*. 2010;24(6):639–648.

24. Snels DG, Hille ET, Gruis NA, et al. Risk of cutaneous malignant melanoma in patients with nonfamilial atypical nevi from a pigmented lesions clinic. *J Am Acad Dermatol*. 1999;40(5 Pt 1):686–693.

25. Farber MJ, Heilman ER, Friedman RJ. Dysplastic nevi. *Dermatol Clin*. 2012;30(3):389–404.

26. Norris W. Case of fungoid disease. *Edinb Med Surg J*. 1820;16:562–565.

27. Clark WH, Jr., Reimer RR, Greene M, et al. Origin of familial malignant melanomas from heritable melanocytic lesions. "The B-K mole syndrome." *Arch Dermatol*. 1978;114(5):732–738.

28. Lynch HT, Frichot BC 3rd, Lynch JF. Familial atypical multiple mole-melanoma syndrome. *J Med Genet*. 1978;15(5):352–356.

29. Begg CB, Orlow I, Hummer AJ, et al. Lifetime risk of melanoma in *CDKN2A* mutation carriers in a population-based sample. *J Natl Cancer Inst*. 2005;97(20):1507–1515.

30. Balch CM, Gershenwald JE, Soong SJ, et al. Final version of 2009 AJCC melanoma staging and classification. *J Clin Oncol*. 2009;27(36):6199–6206.

31. Friedman RJ, Rigel DS, Kopf AW. Early detection of malignant melanoma: the role of physician examination and self-examination of the skin. *CA Cancer J Clin*. 1985;35(3):130–151.

32. Abbasi NR, Shaw HM, Rigel DS, et al. Early diagnosis of cutaneous melanoma: revisiting the ABCD criteria. *JAMA*. 2004;292(22):2771–2776.

33. Thomas L, Tranchand P, Berard F, et al. Semiological value of ABCDE criteria in the diagnosis of cutaneous pigmented tumors. *Dermatology.* 1998;197(1):11–17.

34. MacKie RM, Clinical recognition of early invasive malignant melanoma. *BMJ.* 1990;301(6759):1005–1006.

35. McGovern TW, Litaker MS. Clinical predictors of malignant pigmented lesions. A comparison of the Glasgow seven-point checklist and the American Cancer Society's ABCDs of pigmented lesions. *J Dermatol Surg Oncol.* 1992;18(1):22–26.

36. Grob JJ, Bonerandi JJ. The 'ugly duckling' sign: identification of the common characteristics of nevi in an individual as a basis for melanoma screening. *Arch Dermatol.* 1998;134(1):103–104.

37. Rao BK, Ahn CS. Dermatoscopy for melanoma and pigmented lesions. *Dermatol Clin.* 2012;30(3):413–434.

38. Menzies SW, Bischof L, Talbot H, et al. The performance of SolarScan: an automated dermoscopy image analysis instrument for the diagnosis of primary melanoma. *Arch Dermatol.* 2005;141(11):1388–1396.

39. Menzies SW, Gutenev A, Avramidis M, et al. Short-term digital surface microscopic monitoring of atypical or changing melanocytic lesions. *Arch Dermatol.* 2001;137(12):1583–1589.

40. Carli P, deGiorgi V, Crocetti E, et al. Improvement of malignant/benign ratio in excised melanocytic lesions in the "dermoscopy era": a retrospective study, 1997–2001. *Br J Dermatol.* 2004;150(4):687–692.

41. Carli P, deGiorgi V, Chiarugi A, et al. Addition of dermoscopy to conventional naked-eye examination in melanoma screening: a randomized study. *J Am Acad Dermatol.* 2004;50(5):683–689.

42. Argenziano G, Puig S, Zalaudek I, et al. Dermoscopy improves accuracy of primary care physicians to triage lesions suggestive of skin cancer. *J Clin Oncol.* 2006;24(12):1877–1882.

43. Vestergaard ME, Macaskill P, Holt PE, et al. Dermoscopy compared with naked eye examination for the diagnosis of primary melanoma: a meta-analysis of studies performed in a clinical setting. *Br J Dermatol.* 2008;159(3):669–676.

44. Elbaum M, Kopf AW, Rabinovitz HS, et al. Automatic differentiation of melanoma from melanocytic nevi with multispectral digital dermoscopy: a feasibility study. *J Am Acad Dermatol.* 2001;44(2):207–218.

45. Gutkowicz-Krusin D, Elbaum M, Jacobs A, et al. Precision of automatic measurements of pigmented skin lesion parameters with a MelaFind™ multispectral digital dermoscope. *Melanoma Res.* 2000;10(6):563–570.

46. Monheit G, Cognetta AB, Ferris L, et al. The performance of MelaFind: a prospective multicenter study. *Arch Dermatol.* 2011;147(2):188–194.

Chapter 2

Melanoma Pathology

Carlos Prieto-Granada, Nicole Howe,
and Timothy McCardle

Introduction and Histological Evaluation of Melanocytic Lesions

Melanocytes are neural-crest–derived cells that are vital in the skin homeostasis, being responsible for the protection of the keratinocytes from harmful solar ultraviolet (UV) radiation via the production and transfer of melanin[1]. Normally, melanocytes are located in the basilar layer of the epidermis, following a melanocyte to keratinocyte ratio of approximately 1:10, with considerable variation; depending on the anatomical site and degree of sun exposure. Melanocytic lesions characteristically demonstrate quite protean clinical and pathological presentations and represent a wide spectrum that encompasses an immense variety of patterns, from low-cellularity benign lesions such as lentigo simplex and benign melanocytic nevi, to atypical (dysplastic) melanocytic nevi, and finally to the malignant counterpart: melanoma.

Melanocytic nevi are defined by the nesting of benign melanocytes, and their classification includes several parameters and criteria. The most basic classification, into *junctional, compound,* and *intradermal* nevi, is made taking into consideration the lesion's location in relationship to the skin's microanatomy. Nevi are further subclassified into many different variants, each one with its own set of morphological features; Spitz nevi, blue nevi, and congenital nevi, to name a few. Finally, these lesions are classified according to their clinical behavior and/or hypothetical potential to transform into more aggressive lesions; an example of this concept would be the dysplastic nevus (also known as Clark's nevus) group of lesions.

When evaluating melanocytic lesions under the microscope, one must determine whether it is a benign nevus, an atypical nevus, or a melanoma. This task is not always straightforward, and one should employ stringent and consistent architectural (regarding the overall lesion) and cytological (regarding the individual cells) criteria, some of which criteria are described below. An important factor to consider is clinical information such as the age of the patient and how the lesion presented.

Diagnostic Criteria

Architectural Criteria

- *Symmetry of the lesion from low-power exam*: atypical/malignant lesions are often asymmetrical in shape
- *Architectural distortion of the epidermis*: atypical/malignant lesions frequently exhibit confluent growth with "consumption" and effacement of the rete ridges[2]
- *Presence of upward spread of atypical nevomelanocytes*: atypical/malignant nevomelanocytes involving the superficial layers of the epidermis (pagetoid spread) also favor an atypical/malignant diagnosis

Cytological Criteria

- *Nuclear to cytoplasmic (N:C) ratio*: size of the nuclei when compared to the cytoplasm; increased N:C ratio favors an atypical/malignant diagnosis
- *Nuclear atypia*: which includes variation in size of the nuclei (pleomorphism), irregularity of nuclear membranes, dark nuclei (hyperchromasia), and/or prominent nucleoli or macronucleoli
- *Atypical and deep cellular hyperpigmentation*: deposition of coarse and/or fine cytoplasmic melanin granules is often seen in atypical/malignant lesions
- *Increased mitotic activity* and atypical mitoses

Maturation

Maturation is a particular and important criterion applied to the dermal component, which combines both architectural and cytological features. In benign lesions, the individual nevomelanocytes become smaller, and nests break up into individual cells as they go deeper into the dermis (Figure 2.1, B). This phenomenon is often absent in atypical and malignant lesions.

In summary, with these criteria in mind, when viewing a prototypical benign acquired nevus on low power, a small, symmetrical lesion with sharp, well-defined lateral borders is evident (Figure 2.1, A). The melanocytes are well nested at the dermoepidermal junction, with round- to oval-shaped junctional nests regularly shaped at the tips and sides of the rete ridges. Pagetoid spread is uncommon in benign lesions, unless one is confronted with particular variants such as viewing the center of a Spitz, Reed, or acral nevi, or in cases of traumatized or sunburnt nevi. As one looks toward the base of a benign lesion, the nests become smaller (maturation), and no deep mitoses or pigment are found.

On the other hand, melanomas are quite frequently broad, asymmetrical lesions (Figure 2.1, C, top picture). There are more non-nested than nested melanocytes in melanomas. Those a typical melanocytes that are nested often form irregularly spaced, elongated, and bizarre nests, with involvement of the top of the dermal papillae. As one evaluates the deeper portion of the lesion, there is no evidence of maturation and deep mitoses and pigment may be evident (Figure 2.1C, bottom picture).

One should also be able to recognize and assess the degree of sun damage of the skin surrounding the lesion. An important feature to look for is *solar elastosis,* which refers to the loss of elastic fibers in the dermis due to

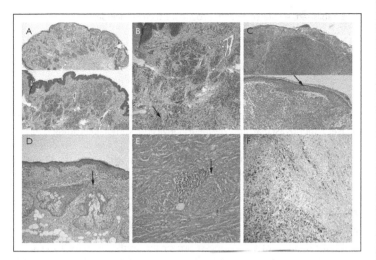

Figure 2.1 Composite image demonstrating representative Hematoxilin and Eosin (H&E) tissue slides from a wide variety of melanocytic proliferations. Both top and bottom images in **A** display low-power views (40X) of banal intradermal nevi to highlight the symmetry of these lesions. The phenomenon of maturation is illustrated in **B** with a medium power view (100X) of an intradermal nevus exhibiting diminution of size of both nests and cells as they progress deep into the lesion. The arrow points out the more mature nevic cells (so-called type C nevus cells). Both top and bottom figures in **C** demonstrate a nodular melanoma. Note the asymmetrical disposition of the expansile nests in the dermis in the low power view (top image, 40X) as well as the lack of maturation and the pagetoid cells (arrow) in the medium power view (bottom, 100X). A case of lentigo maligna melanoma *in situ* is shown in **D**, note the confluence of the intraepidermal melanocytes as well as the adnexal involvement of the sebaceous glands (arrow) (100X). Figure **E** is showing an example of desmoplastic melanoma, composed of bland spindle cells embedded in a fibrotic/myxoid stroma showing lymphoid aggregates and perineural invasion (arrow) (200X). Finally, **F** shows an example of a blue nevus-like melanoma (lower left field of the image) which arose from a pre-existing nevus (right upper field of the picture. (200X).

sun exposure; which produces thick, wrinkled skin clinically, and appears microscopically as a bluish-tinged dermis with loss of the normal pink collagen bundles. Another feature related to excessive sun exposure is *skin atrophy*, which microscopically appears as a markedly thinned epidermis. For further in-depth information about distinctions between benign, atypical and malignant melanocytic lesions one could resort to the excellent melanocytic pathology textbook by Drs. LeBoit and Masi[3] as well as the melanocytic chapter in Dr. Weedon's reference skin pathology textbook[4].

Melanoma Prognostic Factors

Once the diagnosis of melanoma has been made, the pathologist is called on to evaluate many histological features, some of them carrying vital importance in terms of prognostication.

Established, evidence-based[5] prognostic factors include:

- Tumor thickness (Breslow)
- Clark's level
- Presence of ulceration
- Mitotic count (per mm^2), particularly in "thin" lesions (≤1 mm thick)
- Presence of satellite lesions

Other features to evaluate in a melanoma include: tumor subtype, growth phase, lymphovascular and perineural invasion, tumor-infiltrating lymphocytes (host response), and regression. The pathologist must also determine if the melanoma involves the excisional margin, see whether in-transit metastases are present, and measure the size of ulceration if present. The main prognostic factors will be discussed below.

Depth and Level of Invasion

Breslow's Depth/Thickness

Breslow's depth is of the strongest prognostic predictors in melanoma. It is determined using an ocular micrometer to measure the distance in millimeters between the granular layer of the epidermis and the deepest contiguous portion of the tumor[6]. The tumor thickness is directly proportional to the chance of developing recurrent or metastatic melanoma, and it defines the T category in the TNM system:

Tis: *in situ*
T1: <1.0 mm
T2: 1.01–2.0 mm
T3: 2.01–4.0 mm
T4: >4.0 mm

The other distinctions within the the TNM system refer to reginal lymph node involvement (N), and presence of distant metastasis (M). This is more fully discussed in chapter 4.

Clark's Levels

Developed by Dr. Wallace Clark[7], this early method of assessing the depth of the tumor and thus prognosis relies on microanatomical landmarks. (See Figure 2.2.)

Level I: Confined to the epidermis (*in situ*)
Level II: Invasion of papillary dermis
Level III: Invasion of papillary/reticular dermis interface
Level IV: Invasion of the reticular dermis
Level V: Invasion of subcutaneous tissue

After the release of the American Joint Committee on Cancer (AJCC) *Seventh Edition Staging Manual*, the prognostic impact of Clark's level has been greatly diminished in favor of Breslow's tumor thickness[5].

Ulceration

The presence of bona fide tumor-induced ulceration is an adverse prognostic factor, and it modifies the T category from *a* (without ulceration) to

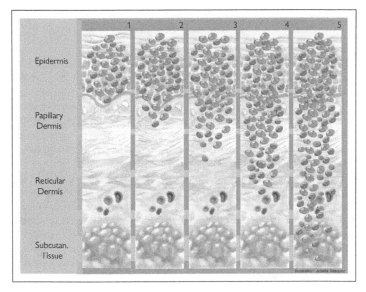

Figure. 2.2 Schematic representation of Clark's anatomical levels:
Level I (1): Confined to the epidermis
Level II (2): Involving the papillary dermis
Level III (3): Filling the papillary dermis and invading deeper into the mid-dermis
Level IV (4): Involving the reticular dermis and the deep vascular plexus
Level V (5): Involving the subcutaneous adipose tissue

b (with ulceration). Tumor-induced ulceration must be distinguished from that product resulting from prior trauma/treatment, and making this distinction is possible via clinical history and specific histopathological changes such as the presence of a fibrinous crust with inflammatory cells in the case of bona fide tumor-induced ulceration. Some pathologists recommend measuring and documenting the ulceration width[8].

Mitotic Count
The mitotic count is performed only in the dermal (invasive) component and is reported in millimeters squared. In the T1 category, mitoses are of vital importance, since the presence of only one mitotic figure changes the category from T1a to T1b (or the presence of ulceration), prompting performance of a sentinel lymph node biopsy[5, 9].

Presence of Satellite Lesions
The somewhat controversial parameter of satellite lesions includes the concepts of microscopic satellites, clinical satellites and in-transit metastatic lesions. The presence of either of the following features in a otherwise lymph node negative melanoma will upstage the patient to N2c[5].

- *Microscopic satellites* are defined as discrete tumor nests greater than 0.05 mm in diameter that are separated from the main body of the tumor by normal reticular dermal collagen or subcutaneous fat by a distance of at least 0.3 mm[10].

- *Clinical satellites (in-transit metastasis)* are lesions that are more than 2 cm from the primary tumor, but not beyond the regional lymph nodes.

Growth Phase

One important concept is that of the growth phases of melanoma, classified into *radial* and *vertical* growth phases (RGP and VGP). However, this particular parameter does not carry prognostic relevance, but it is rather utilized to sub-classify tumors and understand their biology. Melanoma *in situ*, micro-invasive, and thin (<1 mm thick) non-mitogenic melanomas are all examples of RGP. These early forms of melanoma are composed of a tumor clone that has not yet acquired the capacity to invade deeply into the dermis and blood vessels. Thus, during RGP, there is typically little or no metastatic potential, with a resulting good prognosis. Tumors that have developed a VPG, on the other hand, commonly are represented by large, pleomorphic, nodule-like nests in the dermis. These are more expansive than the junctional component and differ cytologically, with frequent mitoses. It is important to recognize that VGP can be detected in early, thin lesions (<1 mm thick), by the presence of a single dermal mitosis[9]. Development of a VGP melanoma clone is linked with a several changes at the molecular level.[11, 12] (See Figure 2.3 for a representation of RGP and VGP.)

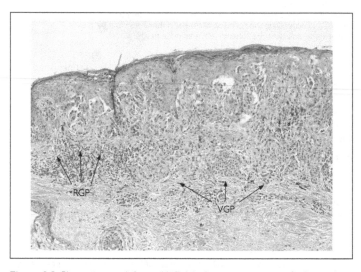

Figure 2.3 Photomicrograph from a H&E slide demonstrating a superficial spreading melanoma with early vertical growth phase (right aspect of the image). The *in situ/radial* growth phase (RGP) component can be seen on the left side of the photomicrograph. Note the distinct nature of the cells composing the vertical growth phase (VGP) (i.e., different clone). Other features of malignancy can be appreciated in this picture, such as pagetoid spread, confluent growth, and cytological atypia (200X).

Melanoma Classification

Currently, melanomas are being classified using a system devised by Dr. Wallace Clark[13], which takes into consideration morphological aspects of the early stages of melanoma (RGP) as well as the tumor location on the body. Clark's classic classification includes four main categories:

- Superficial spreading melanoma (SSM)
- Nodular melanoma (NM)
- Lentigo maligna melanoma (LMM)
- Acral lentiginous melanoma (ALM)

Since the description of this classification more than 30 years ago, great advances have been made in terms of recognizing the different types of mutations present in distinct melanoma groups[14], as well as in understanding the relationship of these melanoma groups to a variety of clinical, pathological, and molecular features. With the advent of revolutionary targeted therapies, mutational characterization of melanomas is vitally important in the modern management of this disease. For these reasons, we favor the new classification proposed by Dr. Boris Bastian, which includes comprehensive clinicopathological and molecular correlations[15]. These clinicopathological features include anatomical location (epithelium associated melanomas versus non-epithelium-associated melanomas) and the pattern of sun damage in the skin where the lesions arise from (chronically sun-damaged skin versus non-chronically sun-damaged skin. Interestingly enough, although it has some modifications and overlap between categories, Clark's original classification remains the foundation and the basis of this new, expanded, and comprehensive melanoma taxonomy.

We will follow this novel classification describing the key clinical, pathological, and molecular findings of each category.

A. Epithelium-associated melanomas:
- Melanomas arising in non-chronically (intermittently) sun-damaged skin (non-CSD): This category includes the SSM, NM, and Spitzoid melanomas
- Melanomas arising in chronically sun-damaged skin (CSD): This category includes LMM and desmoplastic melanoma
- Melanomas arising in glabrous skin: This category includes ALM
- Melanomas arising in mucosa
B. Non-epithelium-associated melanomas:
- Cutaneous (dermal): Includes blue nevus–like melanoma and melanoma arising in a congenital nevus
- Uveal melanoma
- Melanomas of internal organs (Gastrointestinal, Genitourinary, Central nervous system)

Epithelium-Associated Melanomas

Melanomas Arising in Non-chronically (Intermittently) Sun-Damaged Skin

This group includes SSM, nodular melanoma, and Spitzoid melanoma. It is important to mention that the nodular melanoma variant can also arise in chronically sun-damaged (CSD) skin as well as in acral sites. When lesions of this group metastasize, they usually first involve the lymph node basin.

Superficial Spreading Melanoma (SSM)

Superficial spreading melanoma is the most common melanoma subtype and usually affects individuals in the third and sixth decades of life; it tends to present clinically as irregularly pigmented asymmetrical patches or nodules involving the trunk and extremities. The affected patients often bear multiple acquired melanocytic nevi. Since this group of lesions arises in intermittently damaged skin, the features of chronically sun-damaged skin are not encountered.

Histopathologically, SSM are commonly broad, asymmetrical, and fail to mature from top to bottom. Irregular thickening of the epidermis (acanthosis) and effacement of the dermoepidermal junction are evident. A lymphoid and plasma cell infiltrate walls off the base of the lesion. The radial growth phase is characterized by atypical melanocytes with buckshot scatter and pagetoid spread in the epidermis. The melanocytes are large, with abundant pale cytoplasm and vesicular pleomorphic nuclei. They commonly exhibit poorly formed and unevenly spaced nests throughout the epidermis, with a fine dusty pigmentation. The nests may vary in size and shape, becoming elongated, bizarre, or confluent with mitoses. Single melanocytes outnumber the nested ones. See Figure 2.3 for a representation of a SSM.

Key Histopathological Findings of Superficial Spreading Melanoma

- Radial growth phase is present
- "Buckshot" pattern
- Pagetoid spread
- Atypical melanocytes and irregular nests throughout the epidermis
- Prominent dermoepidermal junction activity
- Lichenoid inflammatory infiltrate is common
- Non-nested melanocytes outnumber nested
- Asymmetrical (left to right) with failure to mature (top to bottom)
- Cytologically atypical and mitoses present
- No solar elastosis

Nodular Melanoma (NM)

Nodular melanoma is most often found on the trunk and extremities of males in their fifth or sixth decades. It is characterized by a vertical growth phase. This type of melanoma does not arise in a precursor lesion; therefore, one must ensure there is no evidence of radial growth beyond three rete ridges.

On low power, a symmetrical dermal nodule is evident. There is failure to mature from top to bottom, and deep pigment may be found in the melanocytic nests. Commonly, necrosis is found, as well as a lymphoid-predominant infiltrate walling off the lesion at the base. See Figure 2.1, C for an example of a nodular melanoma.

Key Histopathological Features of Nodular Melanoma
- Dermal nodule with cytological atypia
- Vertical growth phase only
- Junctional activity does not go beyond three rete ridges
- Symmetrical
- Does not mature or disperse towards base of the lesion
- Necrosis common
- Deep pigment in nests possible
- Lymphoid infiltrate frequent at the base
- Plasma cells common in the infiltrate
- Deep mitoses are often present

Molecular Aspects of Superficial Spreading Melanoma and Nodular Melanoma
Importantly, the majority of the lesions classified in this group are characterized by mutations on either *BRAF* (70%) or *NRAS* (15%) genes, with *BRAF* mutations overwhelmingly present in the SSM variant. Over 30 different types of *BRAF* mutations have been described, but *BRAF V600E* seems to be the most prevalent. This mutation is thought to be triggered by UV damage and originates when thymine is substituted with adenine at nucleotide 1799, which results in valine (V) being substituted for by glutamate (E) at codon 600. Secondary genetic alterations in this group include *TERT* mutations as well as *CDKN2A* and *PTEN* deletions. *BRAFV600* mutations lead to uncontrolled tumor cell growth and are the basis for targeted therapy using small molecules with tyrosine kinase inhibition activity, the most well-known one being vemurafenib[15].

Spitzoid Melanoma (SM)
Spitzoid lesions are characteristically very rare, diagnostically challenging, and predominantly encountered in children. They preferentially arise in the head and neck and lower extremities (around the knee), but they can appear anywhere, even in glabrous skin. Clinically, they appear as rapidly growing unpigmented nodules, and there is less of a link with sun exposure. Spitz nevi and spitzoid melanomas can closely resemble each another histologically. Spitzoid melanoma illustrates many of the features of Spitz nevus, including Kamino bodies (eosinophilic globules that are the product of basement membrane degradation), vascular ectasia, and a "raining-down" appearance. However, a diagnosis of melanoma is favored when asymmetry, conspicuous deep mitosis, necrosis, and failure to mature are evident.

Key Histopathological Features of Spitzoid Melanomas
- Similar to Spitz nevus
- Ulceration
- Asymmetry
- Poorly circumscribed

- Pagetoid spread
- Expansile nodule
- Failure to mature
- Impaired maturation
- Deep pigmentation
- Deep "marginal" mitoses

Molecular Aspects of Spitzoid Melanomas

Lesions from this group are characterized by alterations involving a multitude of genes, including *HRAS* mutations and gene fusions involving *ROS1, NTRK1, ALK, RET, BRAF,* and *NTRK3*[16,17].

Melanomas Arising in Chronically Sun-Damaged Skin (CSD)

Lentigo Maligna Melanoma (LMM)

Lentigo maligna melanoma has a predilection for arising in sun-damaged skin of the elderly, typically patients in the seventh decade of life or later, with a clinical history of non-melanoma skin cancer. Clinically, it typically presents with a slow-growing, irregularly pigmented facial patch in the chronically sun-exposed areas of the head, neck, lower arms, and lower legs. Frequently there are areas of regression that appear as white scars or hypopigmented macules. On histological examination, the lesions arise in a background of marked solar elastosis and epidermal atrophy. They are asymmetrical with poorly defined lateral borders, with atypical melanocytes only one cell thick at the dermoepidermal junction—consistent with the fact that the lesions typically extend further than the apparent clinical margin. The rete-ridge pattern is commonly effaced, with poorly nested and confluent multinucleated melanocytes with prominent dendritic processes at the dermoepidermal junction. Although effacement of the rete is common, lentingous epidermal hyperplasia may occur, and lentigo maligna may closely resemble a junctional lentigious nevus or dysplastic nevus. However, a broad junctional lesion on sun-damaged skin is most likely melanoma *in situ*.

Lentigo maligna melanoma lesions often show spindle-shaped atypical melanocytes with hyperchromatic irregular pleomorphic nuclei. Non-nested melanocytes outnumber those that are nested. Nests are unevenly spaced, not limited to the rete tips, and can extend down adnexal structures. Of importance, small biopsies often result in misdiagnosis, as skip areas are common. The false-negative rate of small biopsies has been found to be up to 80%. Therefore, broad thin-shave biopsies are best.

Pigmented actinic keratoses (squamous pre-cancerous lesions) often collide with lentigo maligna melanoma, reiterating the importance of sufficient biopsy size. Both develop in a background of marked solar elastosis with retraction artifact. Actinic melanocytic hyperplasia has an increased number of melanocytes, with mild cytological atypia and hyperchromatic irregular nuclei making margin determination more difficult for surgeons. However, there are no nests, giant cells, or evidence of severe cytological atypia, deep follicular involvement, or pagetoid spread in lesions of actinic melanocytic hyperplasia.

After long-term growth of lentigo maligna, invasive/vertical growth-phase lentigo maligna melanoma may develop. This is marked clinically by a nodule on physical exam. It shares all the histological features of lentigo maligna, with the addition of a vertical growth phase. This can be classified as epithelioid, spindled, or desmoplastic.

Distant spread in this group of lesions presents in equal proportions as satellite, in-transit, lymph node, and distant metastases. See Figure 1D for an example of LMM.

Key Histopathological Features of Lentigo Maligna Melanoma

- Solar elastosis
- Epidermal atrophy
- Broad, asymmetrical lesion
- Skip areas are common
- Spindle-shaped melanocytes
- Predominately junctional growth of atypical melanoctyes
- Cytological atypia
- Dermal mitoses present
- Extends down adnexal structures
- Rete-ridge pattern effaced with giant cells

Molecular Aspects of Lentigo Maligna Melanoma

LMM lesions predominantly exhibit *NRAS* (15%) and *KIT* (10%) mutations, with secondary mutations involving *TERT* and *TP53*. Patients harboring tumors with mutations/amplifications affecting areas from the *KIT* gene that code tyrosine kinase domains (chiefly exons 9, 11, 13, and 17) of the C-KIT/CD117 receptor have shown response to tyrosine kinase inhibitor therapy with Imatinib in recently completed clinical trials[18]. This also applies to the other two melanomas with *KIT* mutations: acral lentiginous melanoma and mucosal melanoma (see ALM and MM discussions below).

Desmoplastic Melanoma (DM)

This group of lesions is encountered in individuals in their seventh decade of life and later, mostly involving the head and neck (35%), trunk (21%), and extremities (27%). Desmoplastic melanomas commonly present as amelanotic nodules or plaques, making diagnosis difficult clinically. As a result, the majority of these lesions are advanced at the time of biopsy.

There are multiple histological variants, and they can be classified as pure DM or mixed DM—the former category applies when the desmoplastic spindle cell component represents more than 90% of the lesion[19]. One variant has abundant pleomorphic cells and hyperchromatic bizarre nuclei throughout sheets of atypical spindle cells. A second form is similar to a scar or dermatofibroma, with thick collagen strands and admixed spindle cells. The last subtype, referred to as *neurotropic melanoma*, often resembles a neurofibroma or neuroma (benign neural lesions). Here, myxoid stroma and cells lacking in melanin pigment are evident. Delicate, spindle-shaped melanocytes are arranged in fascicles in the upper dermis, referred to as *neural transformation*. They illustrate neurotropism, demonstrated by their circumferentially arrangement around nerves. Dense groups of lymphocytes are commonly found scattered in the dermis, with an overlying lentigo maligna melanoma *in situ* in the epidermis in 80% of the cases.

Involvement of lymph nodes in pure DMs is extremely rare (7%). Although distant metastases are rare (usually to lungs), desmoplastic melanomas have a higher rate of recurrence—attributed to perineural invasion and the infiltrative nature of the lesion. Mixed DMs have a higher rate of lymph node involvement. The diagnosis often requires immunohistochemistry, as they closely resemble other spindle cell lesions. Please refer to Figure 1, D for an example of DMM.

Key Histopathological Features of Desmoplastic Melanoma

- Spindle cells
- Lack pigment
- Overlying melanoma *in situ* common
- Perineural involvement
- High rate of recurrence
- Nodular lymphocytic infiltrate
- Neurotropism
- Neural, myxoid, and storiform variants

Molecular Aspects of Desmoplastic Melanoma

The most frequently gene found to be affected in this group of lesions is *NF1* (25-90%)[15, 20]. Recently, the frequency of a polymorphism of the *RET* gene at codon G691S has been shown to be significantly increased in desmoplastic versus conventional melanoma[21].

Melanomas Arising in Glabrous Skin

Acral Lentiginous Melanoma (ALM)

Acral lentiginous melanoma is also more frequently encountered in older patients, in their sixth decade of life or later. It involves the plantar (most commonly the heel) and palmar surfaces and the nail apparatus. This melanoma presents as an irregularly pigmented macule, with one or more nodules if an invasive component is present. Epidermal melanocytes can appear to be benign, as they have only slight upward spread. The rete ridges illustrate lentiginous elongation with atypical melanocytes and mitoses in the basal layer. Marked hyperkeratosis and parakeratosis are evident, with occasional appendageal involvement. There is often conspicuous cytoplasmic retraction. The dermoepidermal junction typically has poorly nested and confluent melanoctyes. Nest formation is a late finding, and invasive tumors more commonly have a spindled vertical growth phase and are less frequently epithelioid.

In addition, subungual melanomas may also occur. This is a rare variant of ALM, most common in Caucasians, with a predilection for the fingers over the toes, especially the thumbs. Clinically, it presents with loss of the nails, melanonychia, or a subungual ulcer or nodule. Histologically, atypical melanocytes are found proliferating from the nail bed. It is most similar to an acral lentiginous melanoma, but desmoplastic, metaplastic, nodular, and superficial spreading variants are possible.

This group of tumors tends to develop satellite, in-transit, and lymph node metastases as the first manifestation of spread.

Key Histopathological Features of Acral Lentiginous Melanoma

- Elongation of rete ridges
- Mild atypia of epidermal melanocytes
- Retraction artifact
- Nuclear atypia
- Involvement of appendages
- Nest formation is late finding
- *In situ* lesions with irregular acanthosis
- Hyperkeratosis and parakeratosis
- Invasive tumors often spindled
- Superficial spreading and nodular variants possible

Molecular Aspects of Acral Lentiginous Melanoma

Mutations involving the *KIT* (15%), *BRAF* (15%), and *NRAS* (15%) genes have been described in this group of melanomas. Amplifications of *TERT* are found as secondary mutations. Interestingly enough, in ALM, molecular alterations such as mutations in the *KIT* gene can be found forming a "field effect," which involves melanocytes away from the tumor that appear morphologically benign[15]. Clinical trials with tyrosine kinase inhibitors were performed in a subset of these tumors[18] (see the preceding discussion on the molecular aspects of LMM).

Melanomas Arising in Mucosa

Melanomas involving the mucosae, tarsal conjunctiva, upper respiratory tract, esophagus, lower gynecological (GYN) tract, and rectum are considered to be mucosal melanomas (MM). These most often arise in the sixth to seventh decades of life and in a precursor lesion with a radial growth phase which closely resembles acral lentiginous melanoma. However, mucosal melanomas can also show nodular, lentigo maligna, and superficial spreading patterns. The most common locations in the head and neck are the sinonasal tract, followed by the oral cavity—more specifically the hard palate, maxillary gingiva, and lips. They present clinically as a pigmented mucosal macule with ulterior nodular growth. Regarding staging and prognosis, Clark and Breslow staging systems are of little utility, particularly in head and neck mucosal melanomas. In 2004, Prasad et al. proposed a classification system that was based on the level of invasion by the melanoma, comprising level 1 (*in situ*), level 2 (superficially invasive), and level 3 melanomas (deeply invasive)[22]. In melanomas of the lower GYN tract, a modified version of the Clark system—the Chung system—was developed (Level 1: Intraepithelial/melanoma *in situ*; Level 2: invasion of <1 mm into dermis/lamina propria; Level 3: invasion 1–2 mm into subepithelial tissue; Level 4: invasion >2 mm into fibrous or fibromuscular tissue; and Level 5: extension into subcutaneous fat)[23]. In GYN tract melanomas, Breslow thickness retains its relevance in terms of prognostication.

Mucosal melanomas have an overall propensity for local recurrence and distant metastases over lymph node metastases.

Key Histopathological Features of Mucosal Melanoma

- On oral, genital, or conjunctival mucosa
- Various growth patterns
- Atypical spindled melanocytes in lamina propria
- Adjacent atypical melanocytic hyperplasia is common
- Variable pigmentation
- Variable desmoplasia

Molecular Aspects of Mucosal Melanoma

Like acral lentiginous melanomas, mucosal melanomas exhibit *KIT* (15%) and *NRAS* (15%) mutations, with *TERT* amplifications being the secondary molecular alterations. Patients harboring tumors with mutations/amplifications affecting areas from the *KIT* gene that code tyrosine kinase domains (chiefly exons 9, 11, 13, and 17) of the C-KIT/CD117 receptor have showed response to tyrosine kinase inhibitor therapy with Imatinib and Sumatinib in recently completed clinical trials. Clinical trials with tyrosine kinase inhibitors were performed in a subset of these tumors (see preceding discussion on molecular aspects of LMM).

Non-Epithelium-Associated Melanomas

Cutaneous (Dermal) Melanomas

Blue Nevus–Like Melanoma (Malignant Blue Nevus)

Blue nevus–like melanoma/malignant blue nevus (BNM) is a *de novo* melanoma that resembles a cellular blue nevus or a melanoma that arises in association with a blue nevus. This rare melanoma variant has been described in all age groups. They commonly present as a blue or black polypoid nodule on the scalp or trunk. Malignant blue nevi have a high rate of mortality, as they are aggressive tumors with a high rate of metastasis, often to lymph nodes, bones, and visceral organs such as lungs and liver. See Figure 1F for an example of a blue nevus-like melanoma (lower left field of the image).

Key Histopathological Features of Blue Nevus–Like Melanoma/Malignant Blue Nevus

Arises from precursor:

- Nodular growth pattern
- Necrosis
- Pleomorphism
- Hyperchromasia
- Nuclear atypia
- Atypical mitoses

Mimicking blue nevus:

- Absence of precursor
- Low power resembles common blue nevus
- Cytological features of melanoma
- Admixed pigment-laden dendritic cells

Molecular Aspects of Blue Nevus–Like Melanoma

These lesions are characterized by mutations involving the *GNAQ* and *GNA11* genes, which are also encountered in uveal melanomas[15].

Ocular Melanomas

Uveal Melanoma

These tumors affect patients in a wide variety of age groups, with the average age being 60 years old. They arise in the posterior and anterior choroid, the ciliary body, and the iris. Clinically, they elicit symptoms such as visual field disturbances and blurred vision. Histopathologically, they present as nodules of plump, spindled and/or epithelioid melanoma cells with macronucleoli. These lesions are notorious for their late metastasis to the liver. They can also metastasize to bones.

In terms of molecular alterations, they share the same mutations present in blue nevus–like melanomas involving the *GNAQ* and *GNA11* genes, with predominance of *GNA11* (90%). Alterations in the *BAP1* gene have been described as secondary mutations[15].

Melanomas of Internal Organs (GI, GU, CNS)

These tumors are extremely rare, and consequently, very little information on them is available. One example is the melanocytoma/melanoma spectrum arising in the central nervous system. This category of tumors is thought to arise from meningeal melanocytes and share many features with uveal and blue nevus–like melanomas, including the most prevalent mutations (*GNAQ* and *GNA11*)[15].

Ancillary Techniques

Histochemistry and Immunohistochemistry

Special stains (histochemical stains) may be used and are exceptionally helpful in certain circumstances, such as when examining an amelanotic or oligomelanotic lesion. Fontanta Masson, a silver histochemical stain, results in a black precipitate with melanin.

Of more importance, immunohistochemical stains utilize antibodies directed toward the antigen of interest. Some immunostains that commonly assist in the diagnosis of melanoma are reviewed in Table 2.1.

Molecular Techniques

A multitude of ancillary molecular techniques are available nowadays that aid with diagnosis and also by directing therapy. The molecular methods that are utilized as diagnostic tools include fluorescence *in situ* hybridization (FISH) and comparative genomic hybridization (CGH). With regard to FISH, there is a commercially available panel of four to five probes that are particularly used in ambiguous melanocytic tumors, whereas CGH provides the pathologist with a panoramic view of the copy gains and losses and also helps define difficult tumors. In terms of guiding the therapeutic options with newly developed targeted therapies in patients with melanomas, tumors now are routinely subjected to mutation analysis for the *BRAF V600* group of mutations.

Table 2.1 Immunostains That Commonly Assist in the Diagnosis of Melanoma

Name	Target	Normal staining	Neoplastic staining	Staining pattern in cells	Staining pattern in lesions	Observations
S-100	Ca2+−binding proteins	Melanocytes Langerhans cells/dendritic cells Sweat glands Myoepithelial cells Chondrocytes Adipose tissue Nerves	Melanoma Nevi Some adnexal tumors Neural tumors	Nuclear and cytoplasmic	Strong and diffuse	Useful in spindle cell lesions, particularly desmoplastic melanomas Sensitive but less specific
SOX-10	SRY-related HMG-box 10 (SOX10) protein (transcription factor)	Melanocytes Nerves	Melanoma Nevi Neural tumors	Nuclear	Diffuse with variable intensity from cell to cell	Useful in spindle cell lesions, particularly desmoplastic melanoma versus scar[25] Sensitive and specific stain
HMB-45	Melanosomal glycoprotein gp100 (Pmel17)	Melanocytes	Most melanomas with the exception of desmoplastic melanomas Nevi **Perivascular epithelioid cell tumor (PEComas)**	Cytoplasmic granular	In nevi, the positivity is present in the superficial portion; the opposite occurs in malignant lesions	Desmoplastic melanomas are negative with HMB-45
Melan-A/Mart-1	Cytoplasmic protein sensitive and specific for melanoma and melanocytic lesions	Melanocytes	Most melanomas with exception of desmoplastic melanomas Nevi PEComas Adrenal neoplasms Ovarian tumors	Cytoplasmic	Strong and diffuse	More sensitive than HMB45

Tyrosinase	Enzyme involved in melanin synthesis and melanosome formation	Melanocytes	Most melanomas with the exception of desmoplastic melanomas; Nevi	Cytoplasmic	Strong and diffuse	
p16[Ink4A]	Cyclin-dependent kinase inhibitor 2A, multiple tumor suppressor 1, tumor suppressor protein coded by the CDKN2A gene	None	50% of sporadic melanomas show alterations; Nevi; High grade squamous lesions of the GYN tract, among others	Cytoplasmic and nuclear	Labeling tends to be lost with tumor progression[12]	
MIB-1 (Ki-67)	Labile, non-histone nuclear protein expressed in G1, S, G2, and M phases of cell cycle	All proliferating cells	Increased staining in malignant neoplasms like melanoma	Nuclear	Deep nuclei positive	More sensitive than mitoses
Phosphohistone protein 3 (PHP3)	Core histone protein that is a major constituent of chromatin; marker of cells in late G2 and M phases	All dividing cells	Increased staining in malignant neoplasms like melanoma	Nuclear and mitotic figures	Mitotic figures positive	
BRAF/VE1	Abnormal protein product of the BRAF V600 mutations	None	BRAF V600 mutated melanomas and nevi; CNS pediatric tumors; Papillary carcinoma of thyroid	Cytoplasmic	Strong and diffuse with good correlation with lesions harboring the mutation[26]	

Other loci that are explored less frequently include specific exons of the *KIT* gene. These mutation analyses are carried out in a variety of platforms, including sequencing (prominently pyrosequencing) and matrix-assisted laser desorption/ionization-time of flight mass spectrometry (MALDI-TOF) types of platforms (SEQUENOM)[24]. With the advent of next-generation sequencing (NGS) techniques, a good number of these tests will be performed in one single platform.

References

1. Lin JY, Fisher DE. Melanocyte biology and skin pigmentation. *Nature*. 2007;445:843–850.

2. Walters RF, Groben PA, Busam K, et al. Consumption of the epidermis: a criterion in the differential diagnosis of melanoma and dysplastic nevi that is associated with increasing breslow depth and ulceration. *Am J Dermatopathol*. 2007;29:527–533.

3. Massi G, LeBoit PE. *Histological diagnosis of nevi and melanoma*. 2nd ed. New York: Springer; 2013.

4. Weedon D. Lentigines, nevi and melanoma. In: Weedon D, Strutton G, Rubin AI. *Weedon's Skin Pathology*. 3rd ed. Churchill Livingstone Elsevier; 2010: 705–756.

5. Balch CM, Gershenwald JE, Soong SJ, et al. Final version of 2009 AJCC melanoma staging and classification. *J Clin Oncol*. 2009;27:6199–6206.

6. Breslow A. Thickness, cross-sectional areas and depth of invasion in the prognosis of cutaneous melanoma. *Ann Surg*. 1970;172:902–908.

7. Clark WH, Jr., From L, Bernardino EA, et al. The histogenesis and biologic behavior of primary human malignant melanomas of the skin. *Cancer Res*. 1969;29:705–727.

8. In 't Hout FE, Haydu LE, Murali R, et al. Prognostic importance of the extent of ulceration in patients with clinically localized cutaneous melanoma. *Ann Surg*. 2012;255:1165–1170.

9. Gimotty PA, Van Belle P, Elder DE, et al. Biologic and prognostic significance of dermal Ki67 expression, mitoses, and tumorigenicity in thin invasive cutaneous melanoma. *J Clin Oncol*. 2005;23:8048–8056.

10. Balch CM. Microscopic satellites around a primary melanoma: another piece of the puzzle in melanoma staging. *Ann Surg Oncol*. 2009;16:1092–1094.

11. Etoh T, Byers HR, Mihm MC, Jr. Integrin expression in malignant melanoma and their role in cell attachment and migration on extracellular matrix proteins. *J Dermatol*. 1992;19:841–846.

12. Strickler AG, Schaefer JT, Slingluff CL, Jr., et al. Immunolabeling for p16, WT1, and Fli-1 in the assignment of growth phase for cutaneous melanomas. *Am J Dermatopathol*. 2014;36:718–722.

13. Clark WH, Jr., Elder DE, Van Horn M. The biologic forms of malignant melanoma. *Hum Pathol*. 1986;17:443–450.

14. Genomic Classification of Cutaneous Melanoma. *Cell*. 2015;161:1681–1696.

15. Bastian BC. The molecular pathology of melanoma: an integrated taxonomy of melanocytic neoplasia. *Annu Rev Pathol*. 2014;9:239–271.

16. Busam KJ, Kutzner H, Cerroni L, et al. Clinical and pathologic findings of Spitz nevi and atypical Spitz tumors with ALK fusions. *Am J Surg Pathol*. 2014;38:925–933.

17. Wiesner T, He J, Yelensky R, et al. Kinase fusions are frequent in Spitz tumours and spitzoid melanomas. *Nat Commun*. 2014;5:3116.

18. Hodi FS, Corless CL, Giobbie-Hurder A, et al. Imatinib for melanomas harboring mutationally activated or amplified KIT arising on mucosal, acral, and chronically sun-damaged skin. *J Clin Oncol*. 2013;31:3182–3190.

19. Chen LL, Jaimes N, Barker CA, et al. Desmoplastic melanoma: a review. *J Am Acad Dermatol*. 2013;68:825–833.

20. Wiesner T, Kiuru M, Scott SN, et al. NF1 Mutations are common in desmoplastic melanoma. *Am J Surg Pathol*. 2015.

21. Narita N, Tanemura A, Murali R, et al. Functional RET G691S polymorphism in cutaneous malignant melanoma. *Oncogene*. 2009;28:3058–3068.

22. Prasad ML, Patel SG, Huvos AG, et al. Primary mucosal melanoma of the head and neck: a proposal for microstaging localized, Stage I (lymph node-negative) tumors. *Cancer*. 2004;100:1657–1664.

23. Chung AF, Woodruff JM, Lewis JL, Jr. Malignant melanoma of the vulva: A report of 44 cases. *Obstet Gynecol*. 1975;45:638–646.

24. Curry JL, Torres-Cabala CA, Tetzlaff MT, et al. Molecular platforms utilized to detect BRAF V600E mutation in melanoma. *Semin Cutan Med Surg*. 2012;31:267–273.

25. Ramos-Herberth FI, Karamchandani J, Kim J, et al. SOX10 immunostaining distinguishes desmoplastic melanoma from excision scar. *J Cutan Pathol*. 2010;37:944–952.

26. Busam KJ, Hedvat C, Pulitzer M, et al. Immunohistochemical analysis of BRAF(V600E) expression of primary and metastatic melanoma and comparison with mutation status and melanocyte differentiation antigens of metastatic lesions. *Am J Surg Pathol*. 2013;37:413–420.

Chapter 3

Biopsy Techniques for Melanoma

Maki Yamamoto and Jonathan S. Zager

Unlike the stable or decreasing incidence of other common malignancies (i.e. prostate, lung, colorectal), the incidence of melanoma in the U.S. has slowly increased at an annual rate of 1.7–2.4% (female and male, respectively).[1] Early diagnosis of melanoma has clear implications for overall survival and is dependent on liberal use of biopsies of suspicious cutaneous lesions.[2] Proper surgical treatment of the primary tumor (determination of margins of excision) and the decision whether or not to surgically evaluate the regional nodal basin when it is clinically negative (by sentinel lymph node biopsy [SLNB]) both rely on precise preoperative assessment of primary tumor pathological factors. Accurate measurement of the Breslow thickness, as well as assessment for the presence of ulceration and the mitotic rate (especially in thin ≤1 mm melanomas), among other primary tumor factors (lymphovascular invasion, satellitosis, regression, histologic subtype), all play a role in the surgical decision-making process.[2] Debate continues regarding the optimal biopsy technique for the accurate diagnosis and initial microstaging of melanoma.[3,4]

An ideal biopsy technique incorporates the following factors: ease of technique, minimal time needed to perform the biopsy and closure, minimal morbidity, acceptable cosmetic result, and most importantly, accurate microstaging of the primary lesion. Initial definitive diagnosis of suspicious cutaneous lesions may involve removing the entire lesion (excisional biopsy) or only a portion of the lesion (incisional biopsy). Incisional biopsies can be performed in several ways, including punch biopsy of a portion of the lesion, elliptical incision of a portion of the lesion with suture closure, or shave biopsy through the lesion. Excisional biopsies are considered to be the gold standard for diagnosing melanoma, and can be accomplished with similar approaches to those listed above, such as a deep scallop shave that encompasses all the lesion along with some underlying dermis, a punch biopsy with a tool that has a diameter bigger than the circumference of the lesion, or excision of the entire lesion and suture closure. While there are clear advantages and disadvantages to each type of biopsy technique, studies looking at recurrence-free, overall, and disease-specific survivals have demonstrated no differences between the various biopsy techniques.[5] The decision with regard to what biopsy technique should be used is at the discretion of the primary care physician or dermatologist, depending on the patient's specific lesion (taking into account both clinical features of the lesion and its anatomical site) and the comfort of the practitioner with the various methods outlined above.

In addition to Breslow thickness (T stage) of the primary melanoma, nodal status is a strong predictor of long-term prognosis and survival.[2] Patients who present with clinically positive nodal disease as evidenced by palpable nodes should have their nodal basin sampled prior to definitive surgical treatment. Fine-needle aspiration (FNA), with or without ultrasound guidance, of suspicious adenopathy should be liberally used.

Excisional Biopsy

Currently, guidelines from the National Comprehensive Cancer Network,[6] the American Academy of Dermatology,[7] and the European Organization of Research and Treatment of Cancer[8] recommend an excisional biopsy with narrow margins, if feasible, for any skin lesions suspected of being melanoma. Excisional biopsy maximizes the likelihood that the entire lesion is submitted to the pathologist. Studies evaluating margins associated with various biopsy techniques note that shave biopsies have the highest risk for a positive deep margin, while punch biopsies show the highest risk for tumor to remain at the peripheral margins, when compared to excisional biopsies.[8,9] Both positive deep or peripheral margins on biopsies may lead to microstaging inaccuracy of the primary tumor—or worse, to a misdiagnosis of the pigmented lesion. Karimpour et al.[10] evaluated 250 patients who underwent incisional biopsies, and found a 21% significant upstaging of their primary lesion upon final excision. Furthermore, 10% were found to be candidates for SLNB only after definitive wide excision was performed.

Excisional biopsies require the most time and technical expertise (see Figure 3.1). After adequate sterilization of the lesion and the surrounding skin, the area is anesthetized with a local anesthetic agent. An elliptical incision (oriented along the lines of potential future excision; i.e., Langer's lines or the longitudinal axis of extremities) is performed with a scalpel, with 1–3 mm margins to encompass the entire lesion. Wider margins are not recommended, as future lymphatic mapping can theoretically be compromised with a larger surgical scar. The resulting defect is closed with sutures prior to applying a sterile dressing. The entire specimen should be sent to an experienced pathologist for careful pathological analysis.

One criticism of excisional biopsies is the possibility of an increased risk of false-negative SLNB due to the disturbance of the lymphatic drainage during an excisional biopsy.[11] One study that may lend some evidence to refute this claim is a study by Gannon et al.[12] who performed a retrospective review of 104 patients who underwent delayed lymphatic mapping and sentinel node biopsy after a previous wide excision or excisional biopsy. The authors showed that they were able to identify the sentinel node in 99% of cases. At a median follow-up of 51 months, none of the 104 patients had evidence of a nodal recurrence in any basin (mapped or unmapped). Hence, this concern regarding the use of excisional biopsy for lesions and that they could

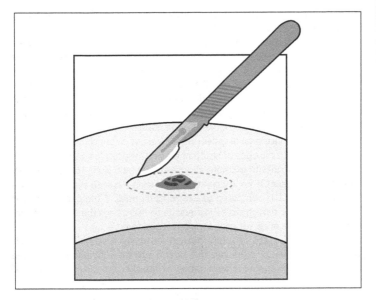

Figure 3.1 Excisional biopsy of melanoma.

lead to interrupted lymphatic drainage or a higher false-negative SLNB seems unfounded.

A potential disadvantage to using excisional biopsies is the theoretical risk patients would require a larger excision at the time of definitive resection in order to excise the old biopsy scar, and any undermining done to close the excisional biopsy while using the appropriate margins for treatment of the melanoma. This, when done on certain anatomical areas of the body like distal extremities (hands, feet) and head and neck, might increase the risk of possible skin graft or flap reconstruction rather than a linear closure of the resulting defect.

In addition, an excision biopsy approach involves a surgical procedure under local anesthesia with suturing for closure that can be time-consuming and difficult in a busy general practitioner's or dermatologist's office. Finally, the cost of an excisional biopsy is higher than that of an incisional biopsy, and may not adequately be reimbursed.

Punch Biopsy

In part due to their perceived disadvantages, and in part because cutaneous lesions are not always recognized as suspicious for melanoma prior to the biopsy procedure,[13,14] excisional biopsies are not always utilized in the diagnosis for melanoma. Three reasons for a subtotal biopsy are lesions in cosmetically or anatomically sensitive areas (e.g., face, hands, feet), larger lesions that are difficult to excise in the office setting, or lesions with a low clinical suspicion for melanoma. In these situations, a punch biopsy can be utilized to biopsy the area of greatest concern, or multiple punches of different areas of a larger lesion can be performed. In small lesions, punch biopsy can potentially remove the entire lesion. Punch biopsies, however, are limited in diameter, with 6–10 mm diameter punches being the largest instruments used in most practices. The primary advantage of punch biopsies is that they extend to the subcutaneous fat and therefore will typically encompass the base of all but the thickest primary tumors. One disadvantage of a punch biopsy is that sampling error may occur with larger lesions, which may lead to misdiagnosis or under-staging. Ng and colleagues[15] looked at the misdiagnosis rate associated with excisional versus incisional biopsies (including shave or punch biopsies). These authors found that the odds of histopathological misdiagnosis were higher with punch biopsies than with excisional biopsies (odds ratio [OR] 16.6, $p < 0.001$). In addition, a higher OR of inaccurate microstaging was seen in punch biopsies (OR 5.1, $p < 0.001$) compared to excisional biopsies. If the punch biopsy is non-diagnostic or thought to be inadequate to microstage the primary lesion, then liberal usage of rebiopsying should be considered.[6]

Punch biopsies are typically performed using a commercially available circular blade, or trephine, and extend into the subcutaneous fat (see Figure 3.2). After adequate sterilization of the skin and injection of a local

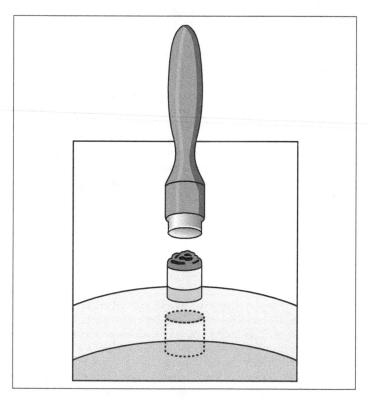

Figure 3.2 Punch biopsy of melanoma.

anesthetic agent, the circular blade is firmly rotated through the skin sur-rounding the area to be biopsied. A subtle decrease in the tension required to pass through the tissue indicates passage into the subcutaneous fat. The specimen is then truncated at this level with a sterile scalpel or scissor. If the lesion is small, this is an ideal technique to encompass the entire lesion. If the lesion is larger, care should be taken to choose the thickest or most clinically suspicious area to be biopsied. The resulting defect can be allowed to heal through secondary intention (especially with very small punches) or closed with one or two simple sutures.

Shave Biopsy

Shave biopsy is the most frequently utilized technique for biopsy of cutane-ous lesions due to its ease of use, excellent cosmetic result, swiftness, low cost, as well as the absence of suturing required.[16–19] Multiple retrospective studies have evaluated the diagnostic accuracy and tumor-staging effective-ness of superficial and deep-shave biopsies (a.k.a. "saucerization"), along with punch biopsies, in relation to excisional biopsies.[14,15,19] In the Ng study,[15] shave biopsies had an OR 2.6 of misdiagnosis of the lesion compared to exci-sional biopsies ($p = 0.02$). Inaccurate microstaging was also more likely in shave biopsies (OR 2.3, $p < 0.01$) than in excisional biopsies. Other studies have concluded that shave biopsies are accurate when determining diagnosis of melanoma as well as the T stage of disease. Ng et al.[20] looked at 145 patients with melanoma and showed superficial and deep shave biopsies had the highest accuracy of true Breslow depth (defined as no change in greatest Breslow depth if there was residual tumor in the wide excision specimen). The authors noted that superficial shave and deep-shave biopsies reflected the thickest Breslow depth before and after wide excision in 93.3% and 91.9% of patients, respectively, compared to punch biopsies where only 80.5% of presurgical biopsies reflected the true thickest Breslow depth. The largest series to date evaluating accurate microstaging by shave biopsy was a retro-spective multicenter study conducted by Zager and colleagues[17] and looking at 600 melanoma patients. The authors showed that T-stage upstaging (from residual tumor) was only present in 3% of melanoma specimens diagnosed by shave biopsy after definitive wide excision was performed. This translated to only a small subset of patients (2%) who required further operative manage-ment (additional margins) after definitive wide excision with upstaging of the T stage. Because of T-stage upstaging due to thicker than expected residual tumor, 1.3% of the 600 patients needed to have a delayed SLNB. The authors concluded that shave biopsy was an acceptable method for diagnosis due to the low percentage of tumor (T stage) upstaging after wide excision, and the even smaller percentage that needed further operative interventions such as additional margins or SLNB.

Martin et al.[21] evaluated 2,164 patients in a multicenter database who underwent biopsy of melanoma either by excisional ($n = 1,130$), incisional ($n = 281$), or shave ($n = 354$) techniques. The authors showed no difference in sentinel node positivity, locoregional recurrence, or disease-free or overall survival. Martires and associates[22] retrospectively evaluated 714 melanoma

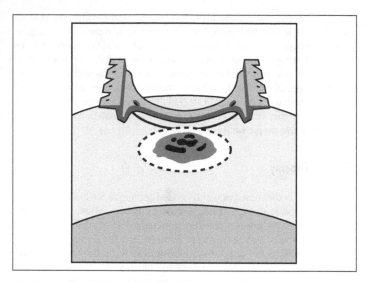

Figure 3.3 Shave biopsy of melanoma.

patients, 171 of whom had a melanoma with a positive deep margin on biopsy (a.k.a. "transected"). Patients with transected melanoma had higher Breslow depth (OR 1.21, $p < 0.001$) than those without transected tumors. Stratified according to stage and Breslow depth, there was no difference in survival rates between transected and non-transected melanomas. Unfortunately, the authors did not stratify according to biopsy technique used.

Shave biopsy is a quick procedure that can easily be performed; making it ideal in a busy office setting. After adequate local anesthetic infiltration and sterilization of the skin, a razor blade/scalpel is applied tangentially to the pigmented lesion, taking care to extend to the expected depth of the lesion to adequately stage the primary tumor depth (see Figure 3.3). Superficial shave biopsies result in a thin specimen of epidermis and upper dermis (<1 mm in depth).[20] Except for melanoma *in situ* or the most superficial Breslow thickness, this technique would be inappropriate to accurately diagnosis and stage melanoma. Most practitioners recommend a deep shave biopsy that would typically extend deeply through the dermis or subcutaneous fat (1–4 mm). Compared to excisional biopsies, deep-shave biopsies leave smaller, more cosmetically appealing scars.[16] With the exception of extremely wide or deep-shave biopsies, there is no need for closure with sutures.

Fine-Needle Aspiration

In addition to accurate microstaging the primary tumor, evaluation of the draining nodal basin(s) is equally important in determining prognosis in melanoma patients. Metastatic spread primarily occurs through the lymphatic system, and the regional nodal basin is the first site of metastases in the overwhelming majority of melanoma patients. Increased tumor burden (microscopic vs. macroscopic) and number of tumor-bearing lymph nodes have demonstrated predictive value in survival.[2] Therefore, the practitioner should have a high suspicion for nodal disease (especially in patients with high-risk melanomas) at the time of the initial clinical evaluation. A thorough physical examination of the regional nodal basins by manual palpation during initial clinical evaluation as well as at subsequent follow-up visits is important to perform in melanoma patients. A high index of suspicion and liberal use of FNA for suspicious regional nodes should be encouraged for all medical professionals who treat melanoma patients. Ultrasound assessment with FNA can be utilized in the cases where there are

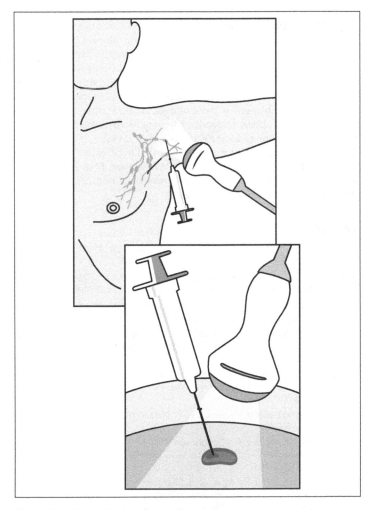

Figure 3.4 Ultrasound-guided fine-needle aspiration.

indeterminate regional nodal findings on physical examination, or when the node is difficult to precisely localize by palpation alone (see Figure 3.4).

Using a syringe or a commercially available aspiration gun, the aspirated material is expelled onto a glass slide and smeared. The slide is then air dried, stained with a rapid Diff-Quik stain, and examined immediately by the cyto-pathologist. In situations of equivocal diagnosis, additional passes can be performed in the same setting. An additional slide is fixed in 95% alcohol and stained using the Papanicolaou method. The material on the aspiration needle can be rinsed and collected for centrifugation and cell block processing.[23]

Conclusion

Diagnosis of melanoma relies on the liberal use of biopsies for suspicious cutaneous lesions by dermatologists, general practitioners, and surgeons. Although excisional biopsy remains the gold standard for diagnosis of melanoma, shave and punch biopsies can also be used. Lesions with low clinical suspicion, larger lesions that may be difficult to fully excise in the office setting, or lesions in a cosmetically or anatomically sensitive area may not be amenable to excisional biopsies. In those settings, punch or shave techniques are viable options and appear to provide adequate microstaging of the primary melanoma. In addition to accurate microstaging and diagnosis of the primary lesion, regional nodal basins should be evaluated by physical examination. In patients with clinical suspicion for nodal involvement, FNA in the clinic or ultrasound with FNA can document the presence of nodal disease and prevent unnecessary sentinel node biopsies.

References

1. Siegel R, Ma J, Zou Z, et al. Cancer statistics, 2014. *CA Cancer J Clin.* 2014;64(1):9–29.

2. Balch CM, Gershenwald JE, Soong SJ, et al. Final version of 2009 AJCC melanoma staging and classification. *J Clin Oncol.* 2009;27(36):6199–6206.

3. Riker AI, Glass F, Perez I, et al. Cutaneous melanoma: methods of biopsy and definitive surgical excision. *Dermatol Ther.* 2005;18(5):387–393.

4. Roses DF, Ackerman AB, Harris MN, et al. Assessment of biopsy techniques and histopathologic interpretations of primary cutaneous malignant melanoma. *Ann Surg.* 1979;189(3):294–297.

5. Mills JK, White I, Diggs B, et al. Effect of biopsy type on outcomes in the treatment of primary cutaneous melanoma. *Am J Surg.* 2013;205(5):585–590; discussion, 590.

6. Coit DG, Andtbacka R, Anker CJ, et al. Melanoma. *J Natl Compr Canc Netw.* 2012;10(3):366–400.

7. Bichakjian CK, Halpern AC, Johnson TM, et al. Guidelines of care for the management of primary cutaneous melanoma. *J Am Acad Dermatol.* 2011;65(5):1032–1047.

8. Garbe C, Peris K, Hauschild A, et al. Diagnosis and treatment of melanoma. European consensus-based interdisciplinary guideline—Update 2012. *Eur J Cancer.* 2012;48(15):2375–2390.

9. Stell VH, Norton HK, Smith KS, et al. Method of biopsy and incidence of positive margins in primary melanoma. *Ann Surg Oncol.* 2007;14(2):893–898.

10. Karimipour DJ, Schwartz JL, Wang TS, et al. Microstaging accuracy after subtotal incisional biopsy of cutaneous melanoma. *J Am Acad Dermatol.* 2005;52(5):798–802.

11. Kelemen PR, Essner R, Foshag LJ, et al. Lymphatic mapping and sentinel lymphadenectomy after wide local excision of primary melanoma. *J Am Coll Surg.* 1999;189(3):247–252.

12. Gannon CJ, Rousseau DL Jr, Ross MI, et al. Accuracy of lymphatic mapping and sentinel lymph node biopsy after previous wide local excision in patients with primary melanoma. *Cancer.* 2006;107(11):2647–2652.

13. Chen SC, Bravata DM, Weil E, et al. A comparison of dermatologists' and primary care physicians' accuracy in diagnosing melanoma: a systematic review. *Arch Dermatol.* 2001;137(12):1627–1634.

14. Tadiparthi S, Panchani S, Iqbal A. Biopsy for malignant melanoma—are we following the guidelines? *Ann R Coll Surg Engl.* 2008;90(4):322–325.

15. Ng JC, Swain S, Dowling JP, et al. The impact of partial biopsy on histopathologic diagnosis of cutaneous melanoma: experience of an Australian tertiary referral service. *Arch Dermatol.* 2010;146(3):234–239.

16. Swanson NA, Lee KK, Gorman A, et al. Biopsy techniques. Diagnosis of melanoma. *Dermatol Clin.* 2002;20(4):677–680.

17. Zager JS, Hochwald SN, Marzban SS, et al. Shave biopsy is a safe and accurate method for the initial evaluation of melanoma. *J Am Coll Surg.* 2011;212(4):454–460; discussion, 460–462.

18. Harrison PV. Good results after shave excision of benign moles. *J Dermatol Surg Oncol.* 1985;11(7):668, 686.

19. Hudson-Peacock MJ, Bishop J, Lawrence CM. Shave excision of benign papular naevocytic naevi. *Br J Plast Surg.* 1995;48(5):318–322.

20. Ng PC, Barzilai DA, Ismail SA, et al. Evaluating invasive cutaneous melanoma: is the initial biopsy representative of the final depth? *J Am Acad Dermatol.* 2003;48(3):420–424.

21. Martin RC 2nd, Scoggins CR, Ross MI, et al. Is incisional biopsy of melanoma harmful? *Am J Surg.* 2005;190(6):913–917.

22. Martires KJ, Nandi T, Honda K, et al. Prognosis of patients with transected melanomas. *Dermatol Surg.* 2013;39(4):605–615.

23. Orell SR, Sterrett GF, and Whitaker D. eds. *Manual and Atlas of Fine Needle Aspiration Cytology*, 3rd ed. London: Churchill Livingstone; 1999.

Chapter 4

Melanoma Staging and Risk Stratification

Prejesh Philips, Emmanuel Gabriel, and Alfredo A. Santillan

Melanoma staging has historically been a dynamic and continuously evolving process. It is based on the existing evidence of factors known to impact prognosis or deliver guided therapy. Over the last few decades, clinical melanoma-staging systems have incorporated a wide array of radiological and biochemical modalities. Staging systems are essential for clinicians to provide prognostic information to patients, develop tailored treatment strategies, and guide the evaluation of clinical trials. Melanoma staging has evolved as more prognostic factors are characterized. In this chapter, we outline the major developments in melanoma staging and their impact on current staging systems and risk stratification.

History of Staging and Prognostic Evaluation for Melanoma

The first attempts to stage melanoma came from Ackerman,[1] based on the knowledge that patients with distant metastases had a poor prognosis. The next major step in staging came from the assessment of microstaging of the primary melanoma site by Petersen et al.[2] in 1962 and took into account dermal invasion. In 1964, McNeer and Dasgupta proposed a simple three-stage system, which incorporated local, nodal, and distant disease burden. This has been recognized as the precursor to the modern Tumor-Node-Metastasis (TNM) staging system. The next significant step was the nearly concurrent work of Clark[3] in 1969, who proposed tumor invasion of the layers of skin as a prognostic marker; and Breslow[4] in 1970, who characterized tumor thickness as a microstaging parameter. Both of these staging systems were subsequently validated[5] as strong prognostic markers. However, the Breslow thickness staging was deemed to be prognostically more predictive[6] and was adapted to the subsequent staging systems.

In 1978, both the American Joint Committee on Cancer (AJCC)[7] and Union Internationale Contre le Cancer (UICC) developed their own staging systems (as did many large-volume centers), leading to an array of conflicting systems that made it harder to interpret contemporary literature. In 1988, a collaborative initiative between the AJCC and UICC developed a uniform staging system based on the well-established TNM system.[8] Over the next two decades, more evidence started accumulating regarding the role of additional major prognostic markers that were not included in the standard TNM staging. These markers included the number of lymph nodes, the presence of tumor ulceration, and the level of lactate dehydrogenase (LDH). Also there was evidence that melanoma thickness was a continuous prognostic variable, such that survival was incrementally worse with increasing thickness, regardless of discrete thickness cut-off values.

Over a period of three years, from 1999 to 2002, experts from various medical specialties, together with representatives from major melanoma treatment centers, assembled and considered all information available in the literature. This group formed the Melanoma Staging Committee and assembled a 17,600-patient database and analyzed the data. The Melanoma Staging Committee proposed significant changes to the prior staging system. These were published in the sixth edition of the AJCC staging manual in 2002.[9] These changes included:

1. Inclusion of tumor ulceration in the Tumor (T) and Node (N) classification,
2. New strata for primary tumor thickness,
3. Number of involved lymph nodes taken as a primary determinant of N staging,
4. Analysis of nodal tumor burden (microscopic vs. macroscopic disease) included as a second determinant of N staging, and
5. Additions to criteria for stage IV disease.

The sixth edition of the AJCC staging system was evidence-based and more comprehensive than the prior melanoma staging systems.

Current AJCC Staging

An updated melanoma staging database containing prospective data on 30,946 patients with stage I, II, and III melanoma and 7,972 patients with stage IV melanoma was analyzed to refine the AJCC staging system. These updates are reflected in the seventh edition of the AJCC staging manual, published in 2009.[10–11] These patients were treated at 17 major medical centers, freestanding cancer centers, or cancer cooperative groups. Independent prognostic factors utilized for risk stratification were considered by the AJCC Melanoma Committee for defining the TNM categories (Table 4.1) and stage groupings (Table 4.2). Survival based on stage has been reported by the AJCC (Figure 4.1).[11]

One fundamental change to the new staging system was the addition of mitotic rate as a criterion for defining T1b primary melanoma. A second was the formal inclusion of immunohistochemical assessment. In addition, consensus was achieved that no lower threshold of tumor burden would be used to define nodal micrometastases. Clark's level was not included in the

Table 4.1 TNM Staging Categories for Cutaneous Melanoma

Classification	Thickness (mm)	Ulceration Status/Mitoses
T		
Tis	NA	NA
T1	≤1.00	a: Without ulceration, and mitosis <1/mm^2 b: With ulceration , or mitoses 1/mm^2
T2	1.01–2.00	a: Without ulceration b: With ulceration
T3	2.01–4.00	a: Without ulceration b: With ulceration
T4	>4.00	a: Without ulceration b: With ulceration
N	Number of Metastatic Nodes	Nodal Metastatic Burden
N0	0	NA
N1	1	a: Micrometastasis* b: Macrometastasis†
N2	2–3	a: Micrometastasis* b: Macrometastasis† c: In-transit metastases/ satellites without metastatic nodes
N3	4 metastatic nodes, or matted nodes, or in-transit metastases/ satellites with metastatic nodes	
M	Site	Serum LDH
M0	No distant metastases	NA
M1a	Distant skin, subcutaneous, or nodal metastases	Normal
M1b	Lung metastases	Normal
M1c	All other visceral metastases	Normal
	Any distant metastasis	Elevated

Abbreviations: NA, not applicable; LDH, lactate dehydrogenase.
*Micrometastases are diagnosed after sentinel lymph node biopsy.
†Macrometastases are defined as clinically detectable nodal metastases confirmed pathologically.

seventh edition. In addition, recent studies by Lee and Cormier that focused on patients with melanoma of unknown primary with metastases to lymph nodes have demonstrated a survival profile similar to (and sometimes more favorable than) survival of patients with regional nodal disease but a known primary melanoma.[12–13] Melanoma from an unknown primary is reflected in the updated seventh edition of the AJCC staging system: metastatic melanoma to the skin, subcutaneous tissue, or lymph nodes with an unknown primary is classified as stage III disease.

Table 4.2 Anatomical Stage Groupings for Cutaneous Melanoma

	Clinical Staging*				Pathological Staging†		
	T	N	M		T	N	M
0	Tis	N0	M0	0	Tis	N0	M0
1A	T1a	N0	M0	1A	T1a	N0	M0
1B	T1b	N0	M0	1B	T1b	N0	M0
	T2a	N0	M0		T2a	N0	M0
2A	T2b	N0	M0	2A	T2b	N0	M0
	T3a	N0	M0		T3a	N0	M0
2B	T3b	N0	M0	2B	T3b	N0	M0
	T4a	N0	M0		T4a	N0	M0
2C	T4b	N0	M0	2C	T4b	N0	M0
3	Any T	N > N0	M0	3A	T1-4a	N1a	M0
					T1-4a	N2a	M0
				IIB	T1-4b	N1a	M0
					T1-4b	N2a	M0
					T1-4a	N1b	M0
					T1-4a	N2b	M0
					T1-4a	N2c	M0
				3C	T1-4b	N1b	M0
					T1-4b	N2b	M0
					T1-4b	N2c	M0
					Any T	N3	M0
4	Any T	Any N	M1	4	Any T	Any N	M1

*Clinical staging includes microstaging of the primary melanoma and clinical/radiological evaluation for metastases. By convention, it should be used after complete excision of the primary melanoma with clinical assessment for regional and distant metastases.
†Pathological staging includes microstaging of the primary melanoma and pathological information about the regional lymph nodes after partial (i.e., sentinel node biopsy) or complete lymphadenectomy. Pathological stage 0 or stage 1A patients are the exception; they do not require pathological evaluation of their lymph nodes.

Prognostic Factors in Localized Melanoma (Stages I and II)

Primary Tumor Thickness (Breslow Thickness)

The most important prognostic factor for localized melanomas is tumor thickness. Numerous studies have validated the clinical significance of the Breslow thickness as an independent prognostic factor.[11] As noted earlier, this is one of the few instances in cancer staging where the depth is an incrementally worse prognostic variable in a continuous manner. Since this is a continuous variable, the AJCC staging system selected the cutoff values of 1.0 mm, 2.0 mm, and 4.0 mm to help classify the T sub-stage. Tumors

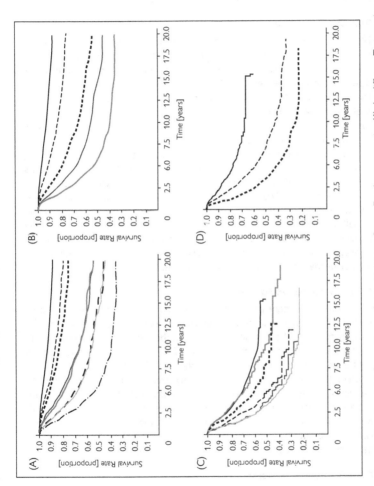

Figure 4.1 Survival curves from the American Joint Committee on Cancer Melanoma Staging Database comparing (A) the different T categories, and (B) the stage groupings for stage 1 and 2 melanoma. For patients with stage 3 disease, survival curves are shown comparing (C) the different N categories and (D) the stage groupings. Reprinted with permission. Balch CM et al: *J Clin Oncol.* 2009;27(36):6199–6206. © American Society of Clinical Oncology. All rights reserved.

measuring 1.0 mm or less in thickness are defined as "thin melanomas" and are prognostically favorable. Tumors measuring more than 4.0 mm in thickness are defined as "thick melanomas" and are prognostically unfavorable. Studies have shown a high correlation between increasing melanoma thicknesses and 10-year melanoma-specific survival. In the seventh edition of the AJCC Melanoma Staging Database, as tumor thickness increased, there was a highly significant decline in 5-year and 10-year survival rates ($P < .0001$)[11].

Tumor Ulceration

Ulceration is defined as an absence of an intact dermis overlying the primary tumor in the presence of immunological host responses on histological evaluation. The negative association of primary melanoma ulceration with worse disease outcome has been studied thoroughly.[14] The presence of primary melanoma ulceration is the third most powerful survival predictor in the analysis for the currently valid AJCC staging system. Although thicker tumors tend to be associated with ulceration, groups have shown that ulceration was still an independent predictor of survival when corrected for tumor thickness as a potential confounding factor. In a population-based study, 5-year survival in patients with ulceration was 66.2% compared to 91.6% in patients with non-ulcerated tumors.[14] Patients with ulcerated melanomas had a twofold higher estimated risk of mortality compared to those with non-ulcerated tumors. Also, the presence of tumor ulceration will upstage a tumor within a shallower depth to that of the next-thicker, non-ulcerated T stage. Why patients with ulcerated melanomas have a worse prognosis is not clear, but ulceration appears to be a phenotypical marker for worse tumor biology and greater propensity for invasion and metastasis.

Primary Tumor Mitotic Rate

A recent independent prognostic factor incorporated into the melanoma staging is the tumor's mitotic rate, which is a measure of proliferation of the primary tumor.[11] The dermal mitotic rate in the vertical growth phase is calculated as the number of mitoses/mm^2. This is typically quantified from a "hot-spot" within the tissue sample, or the area of highest activity.

Over the last few iterations of staging, the mitotic rate was found to be highly predictive of survival. Survival times decline as the mitotic rate increases, especially in thin melanomas. Five-year survival for patients with mitotic rates of 0 mitoses/mm2 was 98.7% compared to 85.1% for those with mitotic rates from 0.1–6.0 mitoses/mm2. Patients with mitotic rates of more than 6 mitoses/mm^2 had a 5-year survival rate of 68.2%.[11]

Clark's Level of Invasion

In 1967 Wallace H. Clark, Jr., characterized melanomas into five histopathological levels of invasion. In Clark's level I lesions, melanoma cells are restricted to the epidermis, constituting an *in situ* melanoma. Level II invasion is characterized by the extension of melanoma cells from the epidermis into the papillary dermis. A tumor with a vertical growth-phase invading throughout the papillary dermis and extending to the junction of the papillary dermis and the reticular dermis is categorized as a level III invasion. The infiltration of reticular dermis collagen fibers by melanoma cells constitutes a level IV invasion. Lastly, level V invasion is categorized by infiltration of melanoma cells from the reticular dermis into the subcutaneous fat.

The Clark levels were the first widely accepted method of microstaging for melanoma. Over time, however, Breslow tumor thickness, ulceration, and mitotic rate replaced Clark's histopathological scheme because the level of invasion was no longer statistically significant when analyzed with these other prognostic factors. Based on current data, mitotic rate has replaced the Clark level of invasion as primary criteria to stage a T1b melanoma. Interestingly, for a subgroup of patients with thin melanomas, level of invasion predicted survival better than did tumor ulceration, while the opposite was true for melanomas thicker than 1.0 mm. In the current staging system, there is no role for Clark's levels. However, if there are no data about the mitotic rate, or if the mitotic rate cannot be accurately assessed in the subgroup of thin melanomas, Clark's level of invasion can be used for prognostic evaluation.

Anatomical Location

The location of a melanoma is also an independent predictor of survival. Axial melanomas are tumors on the trunk, head, and neck. These have a worse prognosis than tumors located on the extremities. Axial melanomas metastasize to distant locations more frequently than do tumors located on the extremities, which spread regionally.[11]

Age

Older patients tend to have thicker melanomas that are more frequently ulcerated. After controlling for confounding risk factors, the age at the time of diagnosis is an independent prognostic factor. A consistent decline in melanoma survival rates with advancing age has been reported.[11] While the reason for this association is not well understood, it has been hypothesized that the senescence of an older patient's immune system and under-treatment of the elderly are contributing factors.

Tumor Regression

There has been considerable debate in literature about the role of tumor regression. Some have advocated the use of this criterion to guide sentinel lymph node (SLN) biopsy. However, in a recent review of tumor regression as a prognostic factor, Burton et al. showed that tumor regression was not statistically significant in predicting nodal metastasis or survival.[15] Therefore, routine use of tumor regression in risk stratification or clinical decision-making is not recommended.

Prognostic Factors: Nodal Metastasis

In patients with lymphatic spread of melanoma, nodal metastasis has been shown to be a very important prognostic marker. It is important to recognize that the use of a synoptic template for histopathological reporting of primary and sentinel nodes increases diagnostic completeness and quality.[16]

Number of Nodal Metastases

The number of nodal metastases has superseded the size of the largest nodal metastasis as the most important prognostic factor for lymphatic metastasis. Multiple studies demonstrated that, in patients with regional metastasis, the number of nodes harboring disease is the most important predictor of survival.[17-20] The current TNM staging reflects this evidence with the use of the number of lymph nodes involved instead of the size of the tumor deposits.

Tumor Burden (Size of Lymph Node Metastasis)

After the number of involved lymph nodes, the size of the lymphatic tumor burden appears to be the next most important criterion. Although this cannot be described in a continuous fashion as is the case with primary tumor depth, the differentiation between microscopic and macroscopic lymphatic disease is important. A *microscopic deposit* is disease that is detected on histological analysis following SLN biopsy or elective lymph node dissection. *Macroscopic disease* refers to disease that is clinically or radiographically detected.

Recently, a large number of stage III patients (3,307) who mainly presented with micro-metastasis identified through SLN biopsy and subsequently underwent lymphadenopathy were analyzed by the AJCC database.[21] As expected, macroscopic disease carried a worse prognosis and nullified the prognostic implication of the primary tumor. Features of the primary tumor (thickness, ulceration, mitotic rate, and location, as described above) were only found to be significant for survival in patients with micrometastasis. Immunohistochemical analysis is now considered acceptable by the AJCC Melanoma Staging Committee to assist in the classification of nodal metastasis. This should be based on at least one melanoma-associated marker such as HMB-45, Melan-A, or MART 1. It is important to note that, unlike criteria used in breast cancer staging, there is no lower threshold of tumor burden used to define nodal micrometastasis. This strongly reflects the consensus that even small amounts of metastatic disease are potentially clinically relevant.

In-Transit Disease and Intralymphatic Metastasis

Currently, patients with in-transit disease or clinically obvious satellite lesions are classified as having N2c disease (stage 3b). Despite some initial suggestion that N2c disease had worse outcomes than advanced lymph node metastasis (N3), current data has shown that patients with in-transit disease have 5-year and 10-year survival rates of 69% and 52%, respectively.[22] These survival rates of patients with N2c in-transit disease appear to be better than the survival rates of patients with nodal disease designated N1b, N2a, and N2b (as shown in Figure 5.1C). Thus for patients with in-transit disease, the current staging system is somewhat counterintuitive, in that these patients are assigned a higher nodal status but have been shown to have better survival.

Prognostic Factors: Distal Metastasis

The presence of distal metastasis is the most important adverse marker of prognosis. Historically, 5-year survival rates of less than 10% have been consistently noted.[23-25]

Lactate Dehydrogenase

The role of lactate dehydrogenase (LDH) as an adverse prognostic marker has been validated repeatedly.[26–28] The reason for this elevation and the exact pattern of elevated LDH isoforms are not clearly characterized. These findings are reflected in the seventh edition AJCC melanoma database analysis. This analysis revealed that 1-year and 2-year survival rates for stage 4 patients with a normal LDH were 65% and 40%, respectively, compared to 32% and 18% in patients with an elevated LDH level.[9] The presence of an elevated LDH level is independent of the site and number of distal metastases.

Site of Distant Metastases

The site of metastasis is the next most important adverse prognostic marker when stage 4 disease is considered. It has been noted that distant skin and subcutaneous tissue as well as distal non-regional lymph nodes has the best survival among stage 4 patients (stage 4a).[10] This subset of patients were classified as M1a in the seventh edition AJCC melanoma staging system. Patients with M1b, stage 4b (metastasis to the lungs) had better prognosis than those with M1c, stage 4c (metastasis to any non-pulmonary visceral site) disease. One-year survival rates among stage 4 patients were found to be 62% for M1a, 53% for M1b, and 33% for M1c melanomas.[10] Five-year survival rates among these patients were approximately 25%, 15%, and 10%, respectively, for M1a, M1b, and M1c.[10]

Number of Distal Metastases

Although the number of distal metastases is not part of the TNM staging system, several independent studies have reported the number of distant metastases to be a relevant prognostic factor.[29,30] However, the practical use of this marker is difficult, because it not only requires the standardization of radiological and clinical techniques but also potentially risks the under- or over-staging of patients. The number of distant metastases remains an important marker, and the future evolution of staging is likely to incorporate this as a prognostic factor.

The Future of Melanoma Staging

Molecular and Immunological Biomarkers

The TNM staging system remains the primary basis of prognosis evaluation. However, among patients with similar anatomical tumor burden, there is often a significant difference in survival rates. This is now increasingly being recognized as a function of varied tumor biology. Therefore, there has been increasing work towards evaluation of molecular and immunological biomarkers. With the development of targeted therapies for melanomas with specific molecular biomarkers, the prognosis of these patients may significantly improve. Recent insights into the genetic and immunological aberrations have initiated a new era of rapidly evolving targeted and immune-based treatments for melanoma. These therapies could serve as additional prognostic and predictive markers to determine a patient's potential for metastatic relapse at time of diagnosis. One of the earlier breakthroughs was the identification of a mutation in exon 15 of BRAF, a signaling molecule in the MAP kinase pathway in cell cycle regulation, in 50–70% of melanomas.[31] This discovery was made clinically relevant with the use of targeted therapy known as Vemurafinib.[32] This targeted therapy is an orally available, small molecule, selective BRAF inhibitor that is approved by the Food and Drug Administration (FDA) for patients with unresectable or metastatic melanoma that tests positive for the BRAF V600E mutation, and has shown promising initial results.

A three-marker immunohistochemistry-based prognostic assay in primary cutaneous melanomas was developed evaluating expression levels of NCOA3 (nuclear receptor coactivator), SPP1 (osteopontin), and RGS1 (regulator of G protein signaling). This was tested in cohort of 395 patients, and expression was then validated in an independent cohort of 141 cases from the German Cancer Registry. The multimarker score was independently predictive of disease specific survival in cohorts, surpassing tumor thickness and ulceration.[33] Recent studies are also focusing on role of PHIP (pleckstrin homology domain-interacting protein) in melanoma progression. Based on recent data, PHIP is a novel marker and mediator of melanoma metastasis.[34] A commmerically available gene expression profile (GEP) assay using a 31-gene signature has been described that in a 217 patient validation set was shown to be an independent prognostic factor.[35] The "immune contexture"—or tumor microenvironment as defined as the type, functional orientation, density, and location of adaptive immune cells within distinct tumor regions—has emerged as an important independent prognosticator. A majority of studies have demonstrated that a high densities of CD3+ T cells, CD8+ cytotoxic T cells, and CD45Ro positive memory T cells are associated with longer disease-free survival and/or improved survival.[36] Immunoscore is based on these findings and is quantified within the center of the tumor and invasive margin. It provides a scoring system helpful in predicting survival in early-stage melanomas.[37] This is being currently evaluated by an international task force for colorectal cancer and melanoma.

These, along with various other molecular profiling strategies, are under evaluation and will probably lead to further evolution of the melanoma staging system and more meaningful prognosis evaluation incorporating existing melanoma therapy.

Prognosis Calculators

With the increasing complexity of staging and the emergence of newer prognostic markers, there is currently a significant interest in the personalization of prognosis evaluation. This would allow for factors specific to the individual patient to be combined with pathological, IHC, and molecular biomarkers to give a composite, multimodal approach in melanoma staging evaluation and prognosis.

Currently, there are two primary online tools that function as prognostic calculators. The first was based on the work of Balch and other collaborators from the AJCC staging committee.[38] The online tool is available to assess prognosis based on individual patient and tumor characteristics. This is available at www.melanomaprognosis.org.

More recently, another independent, validated model from the Sunbelt Melanoma Group was developed. It has been shown to predict prognosis in patients with melanoma staged by SLN biopsy more accurately than the AJCC model, especially in patients with stage 3 disease.[39] This model is available online at www.melanomacalculator.com or as the melanoma calculator application for mobile devices.

With the increasing complexity and the rapidly changing landscape of translational medicine, it is likely that the current staging system will see a paradigm shift towards more inclusive prognostic methodologies that are individualized and can help physicians better construct treatment options.

Summary

The development of an international melanoma staging system has resulted in greater accuracy for prognostication, treatment, and implementation of clinical trials. As new prognostic factors are identified and validated, it may be the case that the staging system may evolve with an increasing complexity that also incorporates patient-specific prognostic factors that also shape individualized melanoma treatment strategies.

References

1. Ackerman LV, Del Regato JA. *Cancer: Diagnosis, Treatment, and Prognosis*, 2nd ed. St. Louis: Mosby; 1954: 1201 p.

2. Petersen NC, Bodenham, DC, Lloyd OC. Malignant melanomas of the skin. A study of the origin, development, aetiology, spread, treatment, and prognosis. *Br J Plast Surg*. 1962;15:97–116.

3. Clark WH Jr., et al. The histogenesis and biologic behavior of primary human malignant melanomas of the skin. *Cancer Res*. 1969;29(3):705–727.

4. Breslow A. Thickness, cross-sectional areas and depth of invasion in the prognosis of cutaneous melanoma. *Ann Surg*. 1970;172(5):902–908.

5. McGovern VJ. The classification of melanoma and its relationship with prognosis. *Pathology*. 1970;2(2):85–98.

6. Balch CM, et al. A multifactorial analysis of melanoma: prognostic histopathological features comparing Clark's and Breslow's staging methods. *Ann Surg*. 1978;188(6):732–742.

7. Beahrs OH, Myers MH, American Joint Committee on Cancer. *Manual for Staging of Cancer*, 2nd ed. Philadelphia: Lippincott; 1983: xvii, 250 p.

8. Beahrs OH, American Joint Committee on Cancer, and American Cancer Society. *Manual for Staging of Cancer*, 3rd ed. Philadelphia: Lippincott; 1988: xix, 292 p.

9. Beahrs OH, et al., American Joint Committee on Cancer, and American Cancer Society. *Manual for Staging of Cancer*, 6th ed. New York: Springer; 2002.

10. Edge SB, et al., American Joint Committee on Cancer, and American Cancer Society. *Manual for staging of cancer*, 7th ed. New York: Springer; 2009.

11. Balch CM, et al. Final version of 2009 AJCC melanoma staging and classification. *J Clin Oncol*. 2009;27(36):6199–6206.

12. Lee CC, et al. Improved survival after lymphadenectomy for nodal metastasis from an unknown primary melanoma. *J Clin Oncol*. 2008;26(4):535–541.

13. Cormier JN, et al. Metastatic melanoma to lymph nodes in patients with unknown primary sites. *Cancer*. 2006;106(9):2012–2020.

14. McGovern VJ, et al. Ulceration and prognosis in cutaneous malignant melanoma. *Histopathology*. 1982;6(4):399–407.

15. Burton AL, et al. Regression does not predict nodal metastasis or survival in patients with cutaneous melanoma. *Am Surg*. 2011;77(8):1009–1013.

16. Haydu LE, et al. Quality of histopathological reporting on melanoma and influence of use of a synoptic template. *Histopathology*. 2010;56(6):768–774.

17. Buzaid AC, Anderson CM. The changing prognosis of melanoma. *Curr Oncol Rep*. 2000;2(4):322–328.

18. Gershenwald JE, Fischer D, Buzaid AC. Clinical classification and staging. *Clin Plast Surg*. 2000;27(3):361–376, viii.

19. White RR, et al. Long-term survival in 2,505 patients with melanoma with regional lymph node metastasis. *Ann Surg*. 2002;235(6):879–887.

20. Balch CM, et al. Final version of the American Joint Committee on Cancer staging system for cutaneous melanoma. *J Clin Oncol*. 2001;19(16):3635–3648.

21. Balch CM, et al. Multivariate analysis of prognostic factors among 2,313 patients with stage III melanoma: comparison of nodal micrometastases versus macrometastases. *J Clin Oncol*. 2010;28(14):2452–2459.

22. Leon P, et al. The prognostic implications of microscopic satellites in patients with clinical stage I melanoma. *Arch Surg*. 1991;126(12):1461–1468.

23. Barth A, Wanek LA, Morton DL. Prognostic factors in 1,521 melanoma patients with distant metastases. *J Am Coll Surg*. 1995;181(3):193–201.

24. Manola J, et al. Prognostic factors in metastatic melanoma: a pooled analysis of Eastern Cooperative Oncology Group trials. *J Clin Oncol*. 2000;18(22):3782–3793.

25. Eton O, et al. Prognostic factors for survival of patients treated systemically for disseminated melanoma. *J Clin Oncol*. 1998;16(3):1103–1111.

26. Bedikian AY, et al. Prognostic factors that determine the long-term survival of patients with unresectable metastatic melanoma. *Cancer Invest*. 2008;26(6):624–633.

27. Keilholz U, et al. Prognostic factors for survival and factors associated with long-term remission in patients with advanced melanoma receiving cytokine-based treatments: second analysis of a randomised EORTC Melanoma Group trial comparing interferon-alpha2a (IFNalpha) and interleukin 2 (IL-2) with or without cisplatin. *Eur J Cancer*. 2002;38(11):1501–1511.

28. Sirott MN, et al. Prognostic factors in patients with metastatic malignant melanoma. A multivariate analysis. *Cancer*. 1993;72(10):3091–3098.

29. Balch CM, Cutaneous melanoma: prognosis and treatment results worldwide. *Semin Surg Oncol*. 1992;8(6):400–414.

30. Staudt M, et al. Determinants of survival in patients with brain metastases from cutaneous melanoma. *Br J Cancer*. 2010;102(8):1213–1218.

31. Davies H, et al. Mutations of the *BRAF* gene in human cancer. *Nature*. 2002;417(6892):949–954.

32. Joseph EW, et al. The RAF inhibitor PLX4032 inhibits ERK signaling and tumor cell proliferation in a V600E *BRAF*-selective manner. *Proc Natl Acad Sci U S A*. Aug 17, 2010;107(33):14903–14908.

33. Kashani-Sabet M, et al. A multimarker prognostic assay for primary cutaneous melanoma. *Clin Cancer Res.* 2009;15(22):6987–6992.

34. De Semir D, et al. Pleckstrin homology domain-interacting protein (PHIP) as a marker and mediator of melanoma metastasis. *Proc Natl Acad Sci U S A.* 2012; 109(18):7067–7072.

35. Gerami, P., et al., Gene expression profiling for molecular staging of cutaneous melanoma in patients undergoing sentinel lymph node biopsy. *J Am Acad Dermatol*, 2015. 72(5): p. 780-5 e3.

36. Fridman WH, et al. The immune contexture in human tumours: impact on clinical outcome. *Nat Rev Cancer.* 2012;12(4):298–306.

37. Pages F, et al. In situ cytotoxic and memory T cells predict outcome in patients with early-stage colorectal cancer. *J Clin Oncol.* 2009;27(35):5944–5951.

38. Soong SJ, et al. Predicting survival outcome of localized melanoma: an electronic prediction tool based on the AJCC Melanoma Database. *Ann Surg Oncol.* 2010;17(8):2006–2014.

39. Callender GG, et al. A novel and accurate computer model of melanoma prognosis for patients staged by sentinel lymph node biopsy: comparison with the American Joint Committee on Cancer model. *J Am Coll Surg.* 2012,214(4): 608–617.

Chapter 5

Surgical Treatment of Melanoma

Matthew P. Doepker and Amod A. Sarnaik

The surgical treatment of localized melanoma has been based on several randomized, prospective clinical trials, as shown in Table 5.1. The treatment of localized, primary tumors has undergone very little change over the last decade. This chapter will review the options of treatment of thin, intermediate, and thick melanomas by specifically examining the size of margin of resection and whether or not consideration of a sentinel lymph node biopsy (SLNB) is recommended.

Diagnosis of Melanoma

The incidence of cutaneous melanoma has been increasing at a faster rate than any other cancer, with an estimated lifetime risk of 1 in 53. An estimated 9,480 will have died from melanoma in the United States in 2013, with over 76,690 cases of invasive melanoma being diagnosed in 2013.[1] Survival is directly related to stage at diagnosis; therefore, early diagnosis is paramount.[2] It is critical to accurately diagnose invasive melanoma in order to offer the appropriate treatment of localized melanoma, which is defined as a definitive wide excision and assessment of regional nodal basins.

The current preferred method for biopsy as recommended by the American Academy of Dermatology is excisional biopsy.[3] Many other biopsy techniques are available, and these include superficial shave biopsy, deep scallop shave biopsy, punch biopsy, and incisional biopsy. Proponents of excisional biopsy state that shave biopsies could lead to inaccurate staging secondary to partial sampling. This would potentially lead to inappropriate widths of margins and potential exclusion of nodal sampling.[3–4] Proponents of shave biopsy tout the ease of the technique, its lack of morbidity, and its time-saving nature. Recently a large, multi-institutional retrospective study analyzed a consecutive series of patients initially diagnosed on shave biopsy to have a Breslow's depth of less than 2 mm to determine the accuracy of microstaging after shave biopsy and its potential impact on definitive surgical treatment. In this study of over 600 patients, recommendations for additional wide excision or SLNB changed in 2% and 1.3% of patients,

Table 5.1 Summary of Prospective Trials Evaluating Surgical Margins

Trial Name	Year of study	No. of patients	Melanoma thickness (cm)	Surgical margins (cm)	Local recurrence (cm)
WHO Intergroup Melanoma Trial	1991	612	≤2	1.0 vs. 3.0	Not assessed
Swedish Melanoma Study Group-1	2000	989	0.8–2.0	2.0 vs. 5.0	Hazard Ratio (HR) 1.02
Intergroup Melanoma Surgical Trial	2001	468	1.0–4.0	2.0 vs. 4.0	70% vs. 77%
Swedish Melanoma Study Group-2	2011	936	>2	2.0 vs. 4.0	Not assessed
HR, hazard ratio					

respectively. Upstaging occurred in less than 3% of the patients.[5] This study demonstrated that practitioners can safely and effectively perform shave biopsy without compromising the definitive management of patients with melanoma.

Surgical Management of Local Disease

The gold standard for treatment of local disease continues to be wide excision, with either 1 cm or 2 cm margins of grossly normal tissue down to, but not including, the muscular fascia. The peripheral margins of excision are measured from the edge of the previous biopsy site or residual pigmentation for all depths of melanoma. Melanoma tumors are characterized based upon depth of invasion from the dermal–epidermal boundary. These are categorized as noninvasive or *in situ* melanoma, or invasive melanoma stratified into thin, intermediate, and thick melanoma groupings, with a corresponding Breslow's thickness of ≤1 mm, 1–4 mm, and >4 mm.

Melanoma *In Situ*

Melanoma *in situ* is a precursor to invasive melanoma, with 5 mm margins being typically used for the surgical resection. Melanoma *in situ* can be removed by wide excision, but there is no randomized, prospective study that has evaluated the optimal surgical margin of excision. The National Comprehensive Cancer Network (NCCN) guidelines recommend a 0.5–1 cm margin.[6] A large prospective study from 2012 evaluated 1,120 cases of melanoma *in situ* treated with Moh's surgery. The authors compared 6 mm to 9 mm margins of excision. In this study, 98.9% of melanomas *in situ* were removed using a 9 mm margin, versus 86% removed using a 6 mm margin.[7] Based on these results, they recommended a 9 mm of normal-appearing skin around the biopsy site. At Moffitt Cancer Center, 0.5 cm is used in areas of cosmetic importance such as the face and neck, or in areas of functionality that would not allow removal of a significant amount of tissue, including the hands or feet. If the melanoma in situ is on the trunk and tissue preservation is not a concern, some surgeons will elect to remove the lesion with a 0.5 cm margin to minimize the length of the resulting scar, while others will use a 1 cm margin to avoid the need for re-excision if there is a microscopic invasive component identified at final pathology.

Invasive Melanoma

Invasive melanomas less than 1 mm thick are characterized as thin melanomas. The incidence of melanoma is increasing, and 70% of new cases diagnosed are thin melanomas.[1] Historically, radical 3–5 cm margins were obtained for all invasive melanomas, including thin melanomas, to lessen the chances of local recurrence. Recent studies have demonstrated that narrower margins are associated with similar recurrence rates.[8] The NCCN guidelines recommend a 1 cm margin of excision for thin melanomas. For melanomas between 1 mm and 2 mm, NCCN recommends a 1–2 cm margin of excision.[6] The 2 cm margin is preferred, but 1 cm is acceptable if a larger margin will interfere with function, distort cosmesis, or necessitate skin grafting for closure. These recommendations are supported by several large, randomized prospective trials, as summarized in Table 5.2.

The World Health Organization (WHO), the Swedish Melanoma Study Group Trial–1, Intergroup Melanoma Trial, and the most recently the Swedish Melanoma Study Group Trial–2 have provided prospectively collected and analyzed data that support the basis for the width of margin excision. These are summarized in Table 5.2. The WHO trial included 612 patients who underwent a 1 cm or 3 cm margin of excision for melanomas with a depth of less than 2 mm. Median follow-up was 90 months. There were four recurrences of out 100 (4%) in patients with thicknesses of 1–2 mm. All the recurrences occurred with 1 cm margins of excision being used. There was no statistical difference between local recurrence (LR), disease-free survival (DFS), or overall survival (OS).[9] This group concluded 1 cm margins were adequate for melanomas less than 2 mm.

Table 5.2 Summary of Recommended Surgical Margins Based on NCCN Guidelines	
Melanoma thickness (mm)	Excision of margin (cm)
Melanoma in situ (MIS)	0.5–1.0
≤1.0	1.0
1.01–2.0	1.0–2.0
2.01–4.0	2.0
>4.0	2.0

The Swedish Melanoma Study Group Trial–1 evaluated 989 patients with melanoma depths of 0.8–2.0 mm treated with margins of 2 or 5 cm. There was no significant difference seen in OS (79% versus 76%, respectively) or recurrence-free survival (71% versus 70%, respectively).[10] The Intergroup Trial looked at 468 patients with melanoma depth between 1 mm and 4 mm who subsequently were assigned 2 cm or 4 cm excision margins. The study evaluated LR at first relapse and at any time for both groups. The LR rate at first relapse and at any time for a 2 cm surgical margin (0.4, 2.1%) was no different when compared to a more radical 4 cm surgical margin (0.9, 2.6%). A trend toward improved OS at 10 years was seen between the two groups, 70% versus 77%, but this was not statistically significant. Interestingly, this study showed 46% of the patients in the 4 cm excision group required a skin graft versus 11% in the 2 cm group, indicating a decrease in morbidity associated with the narrower margin excision.[11]

More recently, the Swedish Melanoma Study Group Trial–2 evaluated 936 patients with tumor thickness greater than 2 mm. The patients were randomized to either 2 cm or 4 cm margins of excision. Preliminary findings have been published in abstract form, and there was no statistical difference in OS or LR between the two groups.[12] A meta-analysis and systematic review was performed to evaluate the optimal excision margins for primary cutaneous melanoma. The meta-analysis showed non-inferiority of 1–2 cm surgical margins compared to 3–5 cm with respect to LR, DFS, and mortality.[13]

For thick melanomas, a tumor depth greater than 4 mm, the current recommendation is wide excision with at least 2 cm margins.[6] While there is no consensus on the optimal width of resection, a multi-institutional, retrospective study reviewed 278 patients with thick primary melanomas over 11 years who had either a 2 cm or greater than 2 cm margin of excision. This study showed no statistical difference in LR, DFS, or OS after a median follow-up of 27 months between the two margin groups.[14] While LR rates have been shown to correlate with increasing melanoma thickness, a margin of resection wider than 2 cm has not been supported by the literature for melanoma of any thickness.

Evaluation and Management of Regional Nodal Disease

The most common initial site of melanoma metastasis is the regional lymph nodes. For a patient presenting with clinically apparent regional nodal metastasis and primary melanoma, distant disease is excluded by cross-sectional whole-body imaging and physical examination. Following this, the standard of care is complete lymphadenectomy of the affected nodal basin as well as wide excision of the primary site. Prior to the advent of sentinel node biopsy, there had been considerable controversy regarding the management of the patient presenting with a primary melanoma at relatively high risk for regional metastasis but without clinically apparent regional disease. Such patients were treated with wide excision, and either a concurrent elective complete lymph node dissection (ELND), or clinical observation followed by a therapeutic lymph node dissection (TLND) at the time of proven regional metastasis. Both methods have significant drawbacks. As only 20% of patients have clinically occult nodal metastasis at the time of the diagnosis of a primary melanoma,[15] most patients undergoing ELND are rendered free of disease with a wide excision alone. Therefore ELND results in unnecessary operative morbidity for the majority of patients (~80%) who do not have clinically occult regional nodal disease. There are also significant disadvantages of delaying complete lymphadenectomy with clinical observation and TLND at the time of recurrence. For the minority of patients (~20%) with clinically occult regional metastases at the time of initial presentation, delaying complete lymphadenectomy may result in metastasis to distant sites prior to recognition of regional metastasis. Additionally, patients who progress with resectable regional disease will by definition have macroscopic disease whose resection is associated with increase operative risk as well as likely recommendation for adjuvant radiation. Both of these can lead to increased morbidity, hospitalization, and costs.

Technique of Sentinel Lymph Node Biopsy

SLNB is a safe and effective way to identify the ~20% of patients who present with primary melanoma with micrometastatic regional metastases for immediate completion lymph node dissection (CLND). SLNB has supplanted ELND for patients who present with clinically node-negative melanoma. The status of the sentinel lymph node is the most important prognostic factor in the diagnosis of melanoma.[6,15] The technique involves identifying the lymph nodes that receive direct lymphatic drainage from the primary melanoma biopsy site. Final pathology, frequently aided by immunohistochemistry, identifies the patients with micrometastases who are then typically recommended for completion lymphadenectomy upon satisfactory healing from the SLNB procedure.

SLNB should be performed at the time of wide excision of the primary tumor. The use of technetium (Tc99)-labeled sulfur colloid and preoperative lymphoscintigraphy has greatly improved the rate of finding the sentinel lymph node. Preoperative lymphoscintography has aided in finding sentinel lymph nodes, especially those that drain to interval basins or minor nodal basins, such as the popliteal or epitrochlear nodal basins, or in-transit nodes such as those seen in the inframammary, latissimus, occipital, trapezius, and twelfth rib regions. One half to 1 mCi of radiocolloid is injected intradermally 1–4 hours before surgery.[16] Some surgeons prefer injection the day before the planned operation to reduce "shine-through" of the radiocolloid, although the utility of doing so has yet to be determined. Intraoperative use of a gamma probe can help localize and plan the incision to further aid in lymph node removal. Other techniques can be added to increase the success of finding the sentinel lymph node. Either methylene blue dye or isosulfan blue 1% dye can be used along with Tc99 sulfur colloid to help visually identify the sentinel lymph node by injecting the dye intradermally in at least four quadrants around the biopsy site. A total volume of 0.5–1.5 mL is sufficient to identify the sentinel lymph nodes. The use of blue dye alone has shown the sentinel node to be identified in 85% of the cases, but the combination of both radiocolloid and blue dye increases the accuracy to over 99%.[16]

Role of Sentinel Node Biopsy

The current NCCN guidelines recommend consideration of SLNB for all patients with clinically negative nodes and a tumor depth of greater than 1 mm. The NCCN guidelines also recommend consideration of SNLB in selected patients with melanoma thickness of 0.76–1 mm with ulceration or mitotic rate greater than or equal to 1 per square mm.[6] It is controversial whether or not an SLNB should be considered for any thin melanoma lesion with a thickness of greater than or equal to 0.76 mm without evidence of ulceration or mitosis. In a large, single institutional study by Han, et al., 271 patients with thin melanoma (≥0.76 mm), who underwent SLNB, were retrospectively reviewed. This study showed that sentinel node metastases were found in 8.4% of thin melanomas ≥0.76 mm, including 5% of ≥0.76 mm T1a melanomas (without ulceration or elevated mitotic rate). The rate of sentinel node metastasis for ulcerated, thin melanomas (T1b) was 13%. Multiple logistical regression analysis showed only ulceration to be a significant predictor of SLN metastasis, while mitotic rate ≥1/mm^2 trended toward significance.[15] From the results of this study, it is reasonable to consider SLNB for all patients with thin melanoma (T1a or T1b) greater than or equal to 0.76 mm in depth.

Faries et al. looked at 357 patients who either had a wide excision followed by SLNB with potential CLND, or wide excision alone with delayed CLND. Patients with a positive SLN would have an early CLND, while the other group would receive a delayed CLND for clinically detected nodal recurrence. There was no significant difference in acute morbidity, but there was a statistically significantly higher rate of lymphedema in the delayed group (20.4% vs. 12.4%). The length of hospital stay was also longer for the delayed group compared to early. These data demonstrate the additional benefits of early completion lymphadenectomy.[17]

The Multicenter Selective Lymphadenectomy Trial–I (MSLT-I) evaluated 1,347 patients with intermediate-thickness melanoma (1.2–3.5 mm), who were randomly assigned to a wide excision and SLN biopsy with potential CLND for a positive sentinel lymph node, or a wide excision and observation of the regional nodal basins, with potential lymphadenectomy for nodal recurrence. At the third interim analysis, there was no difference with respect toward melanoma-specific survival, but improvement was seen in five-year DFS. In the final analysis published in February of 2014, there was no difference between the sentinel lymph node group and the observation group with respect to melanoma-specific survival at 10 years (81.4% and 78.3%). There was improvement in 10-year DFS of 71.3% and 64.7% in favor of the sentinel lymph node group.[18–21]

The final analysis of the MSLT-I trial included 314 patients with thick melanomas, defined as >3.5 mm. Among patients with thick melanomas, the 10-year DFS between the sentinel lymph node group and observation group was 50.7% and 40.5%, respectively. The final analysis concluded that staging with SLNB can provide important prognostic information and identify patients who may benefit from early completion lymphadenectomy.[21]

A large, single institutional study by Gershenwald, et al. reviewed 131 patients who had melanoma greater than 4 mm who underwent lymphatic mapping and SLNB. Lymphatic mapping and SLNB were successful in 96% of the cases. Final analysis showed the SLNB to be positive in 49 patients (39%).[22] This study concluded that SLNB is highly accurate in patients with thick melanoma, and also identified those who would benefit from an early complete lymphadenectomy of the affected nodal basins. The NCCN and American Society of Clinical Oncology/Society of Surgical Oncology ASCO/SSO guidelines recommend consideration of SLNB in these patients as it may provide important staging and prognostic information, along with access to potential adjuvant therapy at an earlier stage.[6, 23]

Interestingly, only about 15–18% of completion lymphadenectomy specimens after SLNB contain additional nodes (i.e., non-sentinel nodes) with metastatic disease.[24–25] The Multicenter Selective Lymphadenectomy Trial II (MSLT-II) will investigate whether a completion lymphadenectomy after a positive sentinel lymph node is warranted, by randomizing patients to either observation of the affected nodal basin or completion lymphadenectomy after a positive sentinel lymph node. It is possible that the conduct of a sentinel node biopsy may allow select patients to avoid completion lymphadenectomy. This trial has reached its accrual goal in 2014 of 1,925 patients and awaits formal survival analysis.

References

1. Siegel R, Naishadham D, Jemal A. Cancer statistics, 2013. *CA Cancer J Clin.* 2012;62:10–29.

2. Balch CM, Gershenwald JE, Soong S, et al. Final Version of 2009 AJCC Melanoma Staging and Classification. *J Clin Oncol.* 2009;27(36):6199–6206.

3. Riker AI, Glass F, Perez I, et al. Cutaneous melanoma: methods of biopsy and definitive surgical excision. *Dermatologic Therapy.* 2005;18:387–393.

4. Roses DF, Ackerman AB, Harris MN, et al. Assessment of biopsy techniques and histopathologic interpretations of primary cutaneous malignant melanoma. *Ann Surg.* 1979;189:294–297.

5. Zager JS, Hochwald SN, Marzban, et al. Shave biopsy is a safe and accurate method for the initial evaluation of melanoma. *J Am Coll Surg.* 2011;4:450–460.

6. National Comprehensive Cancer Network. *NCCN Clinical Practice Guidelines in Oncology (NCCN Guidelines): Melanoma, Version 1. 2013.* Fort Washington, PA: National Comprehensive Cancer Network; 2013. Available at: www.NCCN.org, 2013.

7. Kunishige JH, Brodland DG, Zitelli JA. Surgical margins for melanoma in situ. *J Am Acad Dermatol.* 2012;3:438–444.

8. McKinnon JG, Yu XQ, McCarthy WH, et al. Prognosis for patients with thin cutaneous melanoma: long term survival data from New South Wales Central Cancer Registry and the Sydney Melanoma Unit. *Cancer.* 2003;98:1223–1231.

9. Veronesi U, Cascinelli N, Adamus J, et al. Thin stage I primary cutaneous malignant melanoma. Comparison of excision margin of 1 or 3 cm. *N Engl J Med.* 1988;318:1159–1162.

10. Cohn-Cedermark G, Rurqvist LE, Andersson R, et al. Long term results of a randomized study by the Swedish Melanoma Study on 2 cm versus 5 cm resection margins for patients with cutaneous melanoma with tumor thickness of 0.8–2 mm. *Cancer.* 2000;89:1495–1501.

11. Balch CM, Soong SJ, Smith T, et al. Long term results of a prospective surgical trial comparing 2 cm vs. 4 cm excision margins for 740 patients with 1–4 mm melanomas. *Ann Surg Oncol.* 2001;8:101–108.

12. Gilgren P, Drzewiecki KT, Niin M, et al. Two-cm versus 4-cm surgical excision margins for primary cutaneous melanoma thicker than 2 mm: a randomized multicenter trial. *Lancet.* 2011;378(9803):1635–1642.

13. Haigh PL, DiFronzo LA, McCready DR. Optimal excision margins for primary cutaneous melanoma: systematic review and meta analysis. *Can J Surg.* 2003;46:419–426.

14. Heaton K, Sussman J, Gershenwald J, et al. Surgical margins and prognostic factors in patients with thick (>4 mm) primary melanoma. *Ann Surg Oncol.* 1998;4:322–328.

15. Han D, Yu D, Zhao X, et al. Sentinel node biopsy is indicated for thin melanomas ≥0.76 mm. *Ann Surg Onc.* 2012;19(11) 3335–3342.

16. Morton DL, Thompson JF, Essner R, et al. Validation of the accuracy of intraoperative lymphatic mapping and sentinel lymphadenectomy for early stage melanoma: a multicenter trial. *Ann Surg.* 1999;4:453.

17. Faries MB, Thompson JF, Cochran AJ, et al. The impact on morbidity and length of stay of early versus delayed complete lymphadenectomy in melanoma: results of the Multicenter Selective Lymphadenectomy Trial–1. *Ann Surg Oncol.* 2010;17:3324–3329.

18. Morton DL, Wanek L, Nizze JA, et al. Improved long-term survival after lymphadenectomy of melanoma metastasis to regional nodes. Analysis of prognostic factors in 1134 patients from the John Wayne Cancer Clinic. *Ann Surg.* 1991;214:491–499.

19. Morton DL, Cochran AJ, Thompson JF, et al. Sentinel node biopsy for early-stage melanoma: accuracy and morbidity in MSLT-I, an international multicenter trial. *Ann Surg.* 2005;242:302–311; discussion, 311–313.

20. Morton DL, Thompson JF, Cochran AJ, et al. Sentinel-node biopsy or nodal observation in melanoma. *N Engl J Med.* 2006;355:1307–1317.

21. Morton DL, Thompson JF, Cochran AJ, et al. Final trial report of sentinel-node biopsy versus nodal observation in melanoma. *N Engl J Med.* 2014;370:599–609.

22. Gershenwald JE, Mansfield PF, Lee Je, Ross MI. Role of lymphatic mapping and sentinel lymph node biopsy in patients with thick (>/= 4 mm) primary melanoma. *Ann Surg Onc.* 2000;7:160–165.

23. Wong SL, Balch CM, Hurley P, et al. Sentinel lymph node biopsy for melanoma: American Society of Clinical Oncology and Society of Surgical Oncology joint clinical practice guideline. *J Clin Oncol*. 2012;30(23):2912–2918.

24. Gershenwald JE, Andtbacka RH, Prieto VG, et al. Microscopic tumor burden in sentinel lymph nodes predicts synchronous nonsentinel lymph node involvement in patients with melanoma. *J Clin Oncol*. 2008;26:4296–4303.

25. Vuylsteke RJ, Borgstein PJ, van Leeuwen PA, et al. Sentinel lymph node tumor load: an independent predictor of additional lymph node involvement and survival in melanoma. *Ann Surg Oncol*. 2005;12:440–448.

Chapter 6

Immunotherapy in Melanoma

Maggie Diller and Ragini R. Kudchadkar

Cutaneous melanoma continues to increase in incidence across both genders in the United States[1], and the prognosis for metastatic disease remains poor with a five-year survival of less than 20%.[1] However, improvements in our understanding of the disease and its immune profile have changed our approach to its management. Surgical resection via wide local excision of the primary tumor with or without lymphadenectomy for nodal disease is the cornerstone of therapy for stages I, II, and III. Adjuvant therapy is typically recommended in patients at high risk of recurrence; i.e., those with ulceration of the primary tumor, bulky lymphadenopathy, and so forth. Treatment of stage IV disease has historically centered on the use of dacarbazine and interleukin-2, with only minimal improvements in outcomes and with a risk of significant toxicity. However, the last decade has seen a surge of new immunotherapies that hope to change the landscape of treatment for stage IV disease.

Given its immunogenic nature, research has focused on immunomodulation as a means of treating melanoma in its advanced stages. Monoclonal antibodies targeting specific lymphocyte activation pathways have resulted in enhanced immune function against tumor cells, and in turn, patients have seen improvements in overall survival. Such therapies and their continued evolution carry significant promise in the treatment of advanced disease, both in the adjuvant and the metastatic settings.

Adjuvant Therapy

Interferon

Patients having undergone complete surgical resection but with features indicative of a high risk of recurrence should be offered adjuvant therapy. High-dose interferon alpha2b (HDI) is currently approved for use in the adjuvant setting in patients with stage IIB, IIC, and stage III disease. Results from the Eastern Cooperative Oncology Group (ECOG) and Intergroup trials illustrate the effectiveness of HDI (administered as 20 million International Units/m^2/day intravenously, 5 days per week for 4 weeks, followed by 10 million International Units/m^2/3 times per week subcutaneously) when compared to low-dose interferon-alpha2b (LDI), observation, and GMK (GM2/keyhole limpet hemocyanin vaccine).[2] At 52 months follow-up, HDI demonstrated an improved rate of relapse-free survival (RFS) at 44% compared to both

LDI (40%) and observation (35%).[3] HDI continued to improve RFS compared to observation alone when median follow-up was extended to 12.6 years (Hazard Ratio (HR) 1.38).[2] Additionally, HDI was superior to GMK in both RFS (HR 1.33) and overall survival (HR 1.32).[2] Meta-analysis of these trials confirms statistically significant and durable effects with an overall 17% reduction in recurrence with the use of interferon-alpha2b.[4] While the effects of interferon on overall survival (OS) have not been as conclusive, a recent meta-analysis of 14 randomized controlled trials demonstrated an improvement in both disease-free survival and OS with an HR for death of 0.89.[5]

Identification of specific patient populations most likely to benefit from interferon therapy is paramount, given its associated toxicity profiles and the lack of clear impact on OS. Importantly, tumor load within the lymph node basin as well as ulceration of the primary tumor are independent factors predicting response to adjuvant interferon treatment.[6] Specifically, patients with stage IIb/II-N1 and/or ulcerated tumor show improved RFS, distant-metastasis-free survival, and OS (HRs 0.56–0.69) when treated with interferon, compared to patients with stage III-N2 disease or patients without ulceration.[6,7] This subset analysis is yet to be further validated prospectively.

Though the approval of interferon in the adjuvant setting is for melanoma patients with stage IIB, IIC, and all stage III patients, the number of patients with stage II disease across all studies is limited. Therefore, interferon is generally reserved for patients with higher risk disease.

Pegylated interferon-alpha2b was approved for use as adjuvant therapy in 2011. It is offered to patients with microscopic or gross nodal involvement within 84 days of surgical resection and lymphadenectomy. Pegylated interferon is characterized by a longer half-life and is administered subcutaneously once per week.[8] Like HDI, pegylated interferon demonstrates an improvement in RFS without a clear OS benefit. In the European Organization for Research and Treatment of Cancer (EORTC) 18991 trial, patients receiving pegylated interferon had a median RFS of 3.0 years, versus 2.2 years for observation alone, equating to a 13% reduction in risk of recurrence or death (HR 0.87).[6] With regard to OS, a subset analysis does indicate a benefit for patients with non-palpable lymph nodes and ulceration in the primary tumor, with no benefit observed in patients with palpable lymph nodes.[6] Given that this was a subset analysis, the approval of pegylated interferon is for all patients with stage III disease, not just those with microscopic lymph node involvement and an ulcerated primary tumor.

Due to the toxic effects of high-dose regimens, intermediate dosing has been explored. The Nordic interferon (IFN) trial, a randomized phase III study, reports similar improvements in RFS with intermediate dosing of IFN-alpha2b (administered as 10 million units flat dose subcutaneously, 5 days per week for 4 weeks, followed by 10 million units flat dose subcutaneously, 3 days per week).[9] The majority of side effects reported were mild to moderate, with fatigue reported as the most common symptom.[9] Given the data for intermediate- and low-dose interferon are not as robust as the data for high-dose interferon, high-dose interferon remains the standard of care in the United States.

Overall, interferon should be discussed in all stage III melanoma patients. Though approved in the stage IIB and IIC setting, its use should be more limited in this population, due to the toxicities of treatment and the minimal data in this specific group. However, either observation or enrollment in clinical trials is a valid option in this group, especially in patients who do not want or cannot tolerate interferon toxicities.

Cancer Vaccines

With melanoma's immunogenic properties, vaccination within the adjuvant setting has been explored. Proteins, peptides, and glycolipids specific to melanoma, and most recently, plasmid DNAs encoding these proteins, have been utilized. Results thus far have failed to show improved tumor regression or survival; however, clinical trials are continuing.[7,10] Intratumoral injection of Oncovex[GM-CSF], an oncolytic herpes simplex virus encoded to express granulocyte macrophage colony-stimulating factor (GM-CSF), showed promising results in phase II trials,[11] and phase III studies are currently underway.

Immunomodulators in the Adjuvant Setting

Recent advancements in the treatment of stage IV disease via immunomodulators and targeted therapies have led to the study of these agents in the adjuvant setting as well. Clinical trials investigating ipilimumab, vemurafenib, and dabrafenib in combination with trametinib are in progress. The *BRAF* inhibitor trial results are not yet available, and a trial comparing ipilimumab to interferon recently closed to accrual. One should pay attention to the results of these studies in upcoming years, as they are likely to change the landscape of immunotherapy in melanoma.

Ipilimumab is beneficial in the adjuvant setting, as indicated by early data from the trial EORTC 18071. Patients with stages IIIA/IIIB/IIIC had statistically significant improvements in RFS when compared to placebo (26 vs. 17 months; HR 0.75) in a recent randomized trial.[12] Unfortunately, ipilimumab also resulted in a relatively high rate of toxicity, with 52% of patients discontinuing it due to adverse events (AEs).[12] The most common immune-related AEs were gastrointestinal (16%), hepatic (10.6%), and endocrine (8.5%).[12]

Whether this study changes the standard of care for the use of interferon in the adjuvant setting is unclear. Though experts in melanoma are eager to move beyond interferon as adjuvant therapy due to its toxicity and controversies about its OS benefit, data are insufficient to alter the standard of care at this time. Because the primary endpoint of EORTC 18071 was RFS and the comparator was placebo, this trial did not prove that ipilimumab is better than interferon in RFS. In addition, no OS benefit has been reported thus far with adjuvant ipilimumab. These data, combined with the toxicity rate of 10mg/kg dosing of ipilimumab, is why interferon remains the standard adjuvant treatment option for resected melanoma in the United States as of November 2014. ECOG 1609 results comparing interferon, ipilimumab at 3mg/kg, and ipilimumab at 10mg/kg are eagerly awaited and may represent the first real chance at moving beyond interferon in the adjuvant setting.

Immunotherapies in Advanced Metastatic Melanoma

High-dose interleukin-2 (IL-2) was the primary immunotherapy for treating systemic disease until recently. Cancer vaccination and various immunomodulators that target co-inhibitory molecules such as cytotoxic T-lymphocyte-associated protein 4 (CTLA-4), programmed cell death protein 1 (PD-1), and programmed death ligand 1 (PDL-1) have been added to the armamentarium (Figures 6.1, 6.2). Toxicities for each of the following treatments will be outlined briefly; however, details regarding their management will be given in later sections.

High-Dose Interleukin-2

IL-2 was approved by the Food and Drug Administration (FDA) in 1992 and is currently utilized in treatment of stage IV disease. IL-2 has no direct effect on tumor cells, but rather promotes tumor regression through its ability to stimulate the immune system.[13] IL-2 functions as a cytokine, promoting T-cell activation and proliferation. In the setting of cancer, IL-2 mediates the production of lymphokine-activated killer cells capable of tumor cell lysis and increases the number of cytotoxic T lymphocytes that specifically target tumor cells.[13–15] Studies evaluating the effect of IL-2 in patients with metastatic melanoma report overall response rates of 16–17% in patients given high-dose, bolus IL-2 as a single agent.[13,16] Though response rates are quite low, the real benefit is the small percentage of durable responses that are seen, particularly in patients achieving a complete response after treatment. Of patients treated with high-dose IL-2, approximately 5–10% will become long-term survivors of this disease.

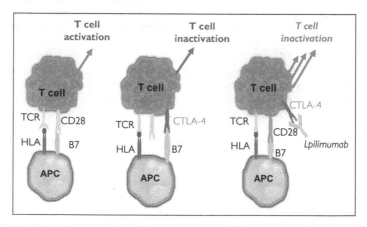

Figure 6.1 Immunomodulator CTLA-4 acts as an immune checkpoint along the pathway of T cell activation. Modified from Weber J. Ipilimumab: controversies in its development, utility and autoimmune adverse events. *Cancer Immunol Immunother.* 2009;58(5):823.

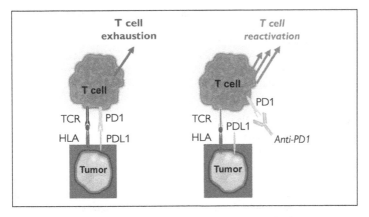

Figure 6.2 Immunomodulator PD-1 is a T cell surface receptor that functions in an inhibitory manner, down-regulating T cells upon activation. Modified from Weber J. Ipilimumab: controversies in its development, utility and autoimmune adverse events. *Cancer Immunol Immunother*. 2009;58(5):823.

Toxicities associated with IL-2 therapy can be significant and can resemble those seen in septic shock, due the vasodilation and capillary leak syndrome that occurs with IL-2.[16] Hypotension is the most frequently reported symptom.[13,16] Additional adverse effects include acute kidney injury and heart arrhythmias, as well as fevers, nausea, vomiting, and diarrhea. There is a definitive mortality rate to this treatment, primarily from unrecognized infection and cardiac arrhythmias. Therefore, patients undergoing IL-2 therapy should be admitted to highly specialized centers where both physicians and nursing staff are trained to manage these specific complications of interleukin treatment. Patients (especially smokers) should undergo both cardiac stress testing and pulmonary function studies prior to initiating treatment with HD-IL-2. It should be noted that despite the severe, acute toxicity of treatment, most adverse effects are reversed within days of treatment termination.[13,16]

Cancer vaccines induce cancer-specific immune responses. Vaccination with gp100 peptide resulted in high levels of circulating melanoma-specific T cells *in vivo*.[17] Schwartzentruber et al. hypothesized that the combination of such a vaccine with a potent T cell stimulator like IL-2 would improve response rates.[18] A randomized phase III trial comparing a combination gp100 peptide vaccine with IL-2 versus IL-2 alone showed significant improvement in overall clinical response (16% vs. 6%), progression-free survival (2.2 vs. 1.6 months), and median OS (17.8 vs. 11.1 months) compared to IL-2 therapy alone.[18] However, treatment with IL-2 alone remains the standard because of the low responses overall from this treatment.

Cancer Vaccines

Many vaccines are being explored, both alone and in combination with other immunotherapies; thus far, no vaccine alone has been shown to improve overall outcomes in stage IV melanoma. Much of the future of vaccine development in melanoma will probably involve combination treatment with other immunotherapies.

Immunomodulators targeting specific T cell receptors are improving outcomes in advanced melanoma. Two principle cell-surface targets include cytotoxic T lymphocyte antigen 4 (CTLA4) and programmed cell-death protein 1 (PD-1). Each functions as a co-inhibitory molecule on the surface of T cells, and their inhibition results in immune activation.

Anti-CTLA4 antibodies

CTLA4 serves as an immune checkpoint along the pathway of T cell activation (Figure 6.1). Stimulation of CTLA4 results in down-regulation of T cells,[19] and its blockade results in tumor regression in patients with melanoma.[20] Ipilimumab (Yervoy®), an anti-CTLA4 monoclonal antibody, was approved for use in patients with advanced melanoma. Randomized controlled trials demonstrate improved OS in patients receiving ipilimumab, both as monotherapy and in combination with vaccination, compared to vaccination alone.[21] The one-year OS for ipilimumab monotherapy was 46%, with a two-year OS of 23% in this pivotal phase III study.[21] Most importantly, ipilimumab has increased the number of long-term survivors with stage IV melanoma with a five-year survival rate of approximately 15–20%.[21]

Many dosing regimens of ipilimumab have been studied. Though higher response rates are seen with the 10 mg/kg dosing, it also has shown a higher toxicity rate. The currently recommended dose for ipilimumab is 3 mg/kg as an intravenous infusion every three weeks, for a total of four doses. The most common toxicities are immune-related and occur in 40% of patients, with 10% reported at grades 3–4; these include: skin rashes, colitis, hepatitis, and hypophysitis.[7] Very few patients have received maintenance ipilimumab every three months beyond the four induction doses; therefore, maintenance is not recommended outside of a clinical trial. For patients who have a durable response to ipilimumab after induction but later progress, re-induction with ipilimumab for four doses can be considered.

Anti-PD-1 and Anti-PD-L1 Antibodies

Like CTLA4, PD-1 is a T cell surface receptor that functions in an inhibitory manner, down-regulating T cells upon activation (Figure 6.2).[22] PD-1 has two primary ligands, PD-L1 and PD-L2.[23,24] PD-L1 is expressed on tumor cells as well as cells within the tumor microenvironment in response to inflammation.[25] Binding of PD-L1 to its receptor, PD-1, inhibits the cytolytic function of tumor-infiltrating lymphocytes and potentiates tumor progression.[26] Antibodies to PD-L1 are currently investigational. Pembrolizumab (Keytruda®), a PD-1 inhibitor, was approved by the FDA in September of 2014 for the treatment-refractory stage IV unresectable melanoma (disease has progressed after ipilimumab and a BRAF inhibitor for BRAF-mutant melanoma). Nivolumab (Bristol-Myers Squibb), a PD1 antibody, is still investigational, but approval for the refractory melanoma population is anticipated.

In patients with treatment-refractory advanced melanoma (disease progressed after ipilimumab and/or a BRAF inhibitor), nivolumab results in a median OS of 16.8 months with one- and two-year survival rates of 62% and

43%, respectively.[27] This study of 107 advanced melanoma patients showed a 31% response rate with nivolumab, with an additional 7% of patients experiencing stable disease lasting six months or longer. In subjects with an objective response, the median duration of response was two years, with 10 of the 33 responders having an ongoing response at the time of publication.[27] In an open-labeled phase III trial of nivolumab in ipilimumab-refractory metastatic melanoma, nivolumab demonstrated a higher objective response rate than chemotherapy (32% vs. 11%).[28] The most frequently reported adverse effects were fatigue, rash, and diarrhea, with grades 3–4 events occurring in 22% of patients.[27] Immune-related AEs were evaluated separately and were primarily related to disorders of the gastrointestinal tract, skin, or endocrinopathies, with grades 3–4 events reported in 5% of patients.[27] Importantly, cumulative toxicities were not reported.[27] Despite being well tolerated overall, pneumonitis has been seen in approximately 3%, and treatment-related deaths have occurred secondary to pneumonitis.

Pembrolizumab also demonstrates similar antitumor effects, with an acceptable safety profile. Importantly, this effect is seen in the treatment-naïve and those refractory to ipilimumab.[28,29] In phase I studies, pembrolizumab produced an objective response rate up to 38% in treatment-naïve individuals, with rates ranging from 26–37% in those refractory to ipilimumab.[29,30] Two doses were evaluated—2 mg/kg and 10 mg/kg—and a dose-related response was not seen. The approved dosage is 2 mg/kg IV every three weeks. The median time to response was 12 weeks, and the median progression-free survival rates were 22 weeks (2 mg/kg cohort) and 14 weeks (10 mg/kg cohort).[29] These data led to the approval of pembrolizumab in the treatment-refractory metastatic melanoma population in 2014. The side effect profile for pembrolizumab was generally mild, with grade 3 or 4 AEs in only 12% of patients, the most common of which was fatigue. Immune-related AEs occurred in 6% and included hepatitis, colitis, rash, and pneumonitis. Most were managed with treatment interruption and corticosteroid treatment.[29] Though these agents have been described as very well tolerated overall, deaths related to pneumonitis have occurred, with the overall rate of pneumonitis being 3% in most studies of either agent.

A recent phase 1 trial reports similar outcomes regarding response rates in patients receiving anti-PD-L1, with an objective response rate of 17%, half of whom exhibited durable responses at one-year follow-up.[31] Additionally, toxicity profiles may be improved compared to other therapies, with only 9% of AEs reported as grades 3–4.[31] Immune-related AEs were similar to those for nivolumab and classified as grade 1 or 2; these included rash, hypothyroidism, and hepatitis.[31]

Combination Therapies

The question of sequencing of immunotherapies has yet to be answered. If high-dose interleukin is to be considered, it is probably best used early in the treatment course. HD IL-2 candidates are typically young, with minimal comorbidities and low disease volume. There are some retrospective data that suggest the response rate to immunotherapy may be lower in the post-BRAF inhibitor setting. Often because of these data and the durability of responses of immune treatments, immunotherapy is typically given before targeted *BRAF* inhibitors. Ipilimumab is typically the front-line immunotherapy for metastatic melanoma patients, especially given that HD IL-2 is not an option for the majority of melanoma patients. Randomized trials of sequencing of different immunotherapies and targeted therapies are underway.

Combination therapy with ipilimumab and nivolumab was recently studied, with promising results. Nivolumab and ipilimumab were administered concurrently every three weeks for four doses, followed by nivolumab alone for four doses. The concurrent regimen was then repeated for patients showing clinical response. Additionally, a sequenced regimen was assessed in which nivolumab was administered in patients previously treated with ipilimumab. Within the concurrent treatment group, objective response rates were 40%, with the majority of responders exhibiting a greater than 80% reduction in tumor burden.[32] Of the sequenced-treatment group, response rates were 20%.[32] Importantly, patients who had been ipilimumab-refractory also responded to subsequent treatment with nivolumab.[32] Responses to combined therapy were varied but overall durable, including the patients who terminated treatment early due to AEs (duration of response ranged from 6–72 weeks).[32]

Biomarkers

With the introduction of immunomodulators as treatment for advanced stage III and IV disease, the identification of biomarkers becomes increasingly important in their potential to predict who will respond to therapy and in individualizing combination treatments. With respect to ipilimumab, several small-cohort studies have identified patterns of receptor expression on T cells that correlate with improved response to therapy. For example, maintained expression of the inducible costimulator (ICOS) on the surface CD4+ T cells is associated with enhanced benefit from ipilimumab therapy.[33]

Programmed death-ligand 1 (PD-L1) expression on tumor cells was initially associated with an ability to predict response to therapy with nivolumab.[34] However, PD-L1 expression is highly variable and depends on the tumor microenvironment and the surrounding cytokine milieu.[35] As such, additional studies are needed to clarify its predictive value, and it should not currently be used to predict treatment response in melanoma.

Toxicity Management

Interferon

IFN toxicities affect multiple organ systems and can be both dose and duration dependent and independent.[36] Neuropsychiatric symptoms, hepatotoxicity, thyroid disturbances, and vitiligo are the most common side effects noted.

Depression is the most frequently reported neuropsychiatric AE.[36] Patients may be given prophylactic antidepressants with selective serotonin-reuptake inhibitors (SSRIs), and those with mild to moderate symptoms for more than seven days should also initiate pharmacological therapy.[36] Interferon should be avoided in subjects with true psychiatric conditions such as schizophrenia and bipolar disorder. Consideration of counseling and supportive care through social work, psychology, or psychiatry should be considered in patients experiencing any neuropsychiatric symptoms. Interferon should be discontinued in the event of suicidal thoughts or psychosis.

Development of thyroiditis and/or hypothyroidism can occur both during and after interferon treatment. Patients should be counseled that the development of hypothyroidism may be permanent and not resolve after discontinuation of therapy. Thyroid function should be monitored monthly during treatment and periodically after treatment. Patients who are status post–neck surgery and/or radiation are at higher risk.

Asymptomatic and mild elevation in liver function studies including alanine aminotransferase (ALT) and aspartate aminotransferase (AST) are common in IFN therapy; however, fatal hepatic failure has occurred.[36] Liver function tests (LFTs) are therefore assessed at baseline, weekly during induction, then monthly during maintenance. Should LFTs increase more than five times the upper limit of normal, IFN should be held, and restarted once dosage of IFN has been adjusted and patient assessment for alcohol consumption and hepatitis B/C has been performed.[36]

Interferon alpha is known to exacerbate autoimmune disorders, especially of the thyroid and skin. Interestingly, autoimmune induction is associated with improved IFN efficacy and is an independent predictor of RFS.[36–38] The thyroid disorders most frequently encountered include hypothyroidism, hyperthyroidism, and thyroiditis. Typically, manifestations of thyroid disturbances are detected within 3–12 months; however, they can occur after completion of therapy.[36] Thyroid function tests should be performed prior to therapy. Should patients develop hypothyroidism, levothyroxine should be administered.[39] Conversely, patients developing hyperthyroidism should be given antithyroid medications.[36,39]

Vitiligo manifests as a side effect of IFN therapy, usually appearing within 3 and 12 months after initiation of treatment.[38] As stated above, vitiligo is associated with autoimmunity, and its appearance in melanoma patients carries a favorable prognosis. Patients should be counseled that this can occur and is likely to be permanent.

Typical side effects of fevers, chills, headaches, and myalgia should be managed symptomatically with nonsteroidal anti-inflammatory drugs (NSAIDs) or acetaminophen. Dose reductions can be helpful in improving symptoms and maintaining quality of life while the patient is on therapy. Daily intravenous hydration during induction can also help manage these symptoms. Other, rarer, side effects include peripheral neuropathy and retinopathy. Patients with any eye or vision complaints should be evaluated by an ophthalmologist. Interferon should be discontinued if retinopathy develops.

Interleukin-2

The toxic effects of IL-2 therapy are significant and probably derive from its activity as a cytokine and potent immunostimulator. Important side effects include hypotension, cardiac arrhythmias, acute respiratory distress syndrome (ARDS) and respiratory failure, mental status changes, hyperbili-rubinemia, and elevated creatinine.[13,16] If mild to moderate, most side effects will resolve within three or four days after discontinuing treatment.[13] Death from treatment-related toxicity, however, did occur in 1–2% of patients enrolled in earlier studies, the majority of which were related to sepsis.[16,13] Interleukin should only be administered at a highly specialized facility by expe-rienced physicians and nursing staff.

Management of severe toxicity largely involves discontinuation of treat-ment. Additionally, due to the early complications associated with sepsis, anti-biotic prophylaxis is administered to all patients undergoing IL-2 therapy.[16] Probably the most important factor in preventing unwanted AEs is patient selection. Routine screening with exercise or thallium stress tests and pulmo-nary function studies should be performed on all patients, eliminating those with preexisting cardiopulmonary disease.[16]

Monoclonal Antibodies

The use of monoclonal antibodies for immune modulation has resulted in a specific subset of AEs, termed "immune-related AEs" or irAEs.[40] T cell activa-tion via binding of these antibodies leads to increased cytokine release and recognition of self-antigens, probably causing many of these effects.[40,41] While most are characterized as mild to moderate, severe irAEs can develop, and early recognition and treatment are paramount in order to avoid long-lasting effects.

Immune-related AEs secondary to ipilimumab develop in a predictable time pattern, with skin-related AEs arising after 2–3 weeks, gastrointesti-nal (GI) and hepatic AEs after 6–7 weeks, and endocrine-related AEs after 9 weeks.[40] Algorithms exist for managing severe irAEs.[42] For AEs requiring high-dose steroids, ipilimumab or the PD-1 antibodies should be permanently discontinued. Management of the most common immune-related AEs will be discussed here.

Management of diarrhea and enterocolitis is critical to the safe administra-tion of ipilimumab. If ipilimumab-induced colitis is not treated appropriately, perforation and death can occur. Initial management of grade 1 or 2 diarrhea is symptomatic with the use of agents such as Imodium. If the diarrhea wors-ens or is bloody, further work-up is warranted. Other causes of diarrhea such as medication-induced diarrhea, gastroenteritis, and infectious diarrhea (both viral and bacterial) should be eliminated. If the diagnosis is unclear, endos-copy can be used. In ipilimumab-induced colitis, patchy ulcers are often visual-ized, and biopsy reveals a lymphocytic infiltrate within the colonic mucosa. Hospital admission should be considered for any cases of grade 3 or 4 diar-rhea. Steroids should be promptly administered at 1mg/kg as well as intra-venous (IV) hydration and bowel rest. For patients with refractory symptoms despite high-dose steroids for five days, infliximab at 5mg/kg as a single dose should be administered. It is rare to ever require more than one dose of inf-liximab. Steroids should be tapered over four to six weeks once symptoms of colitis have resolved. For patients who are unable to tolerate the steroid taper due to recurrent diarrhea, infliximab should be considered.

Hepatotoxicity has been noted in approximately 5% of patients receiving ipilimumab. LFTs should be monitored every three weeks during treatment. One should note that liver tests can increase quickly, fluctuate, and occasionally resolve without intervention. If the levels elevate greater than two times baseline, monitoring of liver tests every three days is indicated. Imaging should be used to rule out other causes. If serum liver tests are greater than eight times baseline, ipilimumab should be discontinued and steroids should be initiated at 1 mg/kg with a 4–6-week taper. If steroid-refractory, the addition of mycophenolate (1 gram PO BID) can be considered.

Hypophysitis is another life-threatening complication of ipilimumab and PD-1 antibodies. Patients may present with just fatigue; however, adrenal crisis can occur with hypotension, dehydration, and electrolyte abnormalities. Rare presentations include headache with peripheral vision loss secondary to inflammation in the pituitary gland impinging on the optic chiasm. Treatment with prednisone 1 mg/kg, thyroid replacement, and testosterone replacement in men are indicated. Patients should be cautioned that lifelong replacement may be necessary.

Dermatitis is typically non–life-threatening but can have an impact on the quality of life of many patients. Patients typically present with a maculopapular, erythematous, pruritic rash. Supportive measures such as moisturizers, topical steroids, as well as oral anti-pruritic medications may be used. Steroids should only be used for refractory, severe cases.

Pneumonitis is a rare event with ipilimumab, occurring in less than 1% of patients; however, pneumonitis is the severest AE seen with PD-1 antibodies. Patients often present with asymptomatic pneumonitis seen on computed tomography (CT) scan. Patients with new shortness of breath, hypoxia, or cough should obtain a CT of the chest to evaluate for pneumonitis. High-dose steroids with prolonged 4–6-week taper should be used for symptomatic patients. Bronchoscopy can be considered when the diagnosis is unclear and to rule out other causes of pulmonary symptoms such as pneumonia.

Conclusion

Overall, immune therapies have revolutionized the treatment of metastatic melanoma, and more patients are now long-term survivors of this disease. Questions still remain regarding the best sequencing and combination of treatments. Additionally, studies are underway to identify biomarkers that may serve as predictors of response and help further guide and individualize therapy. With regard to adjuvant treatment, interferon remains the standard of care. However, given the impact of immunomodulation on stage IV disease, and early studies suggesting the efficacy of such medications as ipilimumab as adjuvant therapy, results from ongoing trials may change the way we treat patients in the adjuvant setting. Toxicities for the various medications can be expansive. Early recognition and management of AEs are key to the safe and effective use of all therapies and in preventing long-term morbidity and mortality.

References

1. Siegel R, Ma J, Zou Z, et al. Cancer statistics, 2014. *CA Cancer J Clin.* 2014;64(1):9–29.

2. Kirkwood JM, Manola J, Ibrahim J, et al. A pooled analysis of Eastern Cooperative Oncology Group and Intergroup trials of adjuvant high-dose interferon for melanoma. *Clin Cancer Res.* 2004;10(5):1670–1677.

3. Kirkwood JM, Ibrahim JG, Sondak VK, et al. High- and low-dose interferon alpha-2b in high-risk melanoma: first analysis of Intergroup trial E1690/S9111/C9190. *J Clin Oncol.* 2000;18(12):2444–2458.

4. Wheatley K, Ives N, Hancock B, et al. Does adjuvant interferon-alpha for high-risk melanoma provide a worthwhile benefit? A meta-analysis of the randomised trials. *Cancer Treat Rev.* 2003;29(4):241–252.

5. Mocellin S, Pasquali S, Rossi CR, et al. Interferon alpha adjuvant therapy in patients with high-risk melanoma: a systematic review and meta-analysis. *J Natl Cancer Inst.* 2010;102(7):493–501.

6. Eggermont AMM, Suciu S, Testori A, et al. Long-term results of the randomized phase III trial EORTC 18991 of adjuvant therapy with pegylated interferon alpha-2b versus observation in resected stage III melanoma. *J Clin Oncol.* 2012;30(31):3801–3808.

7. Eggermont AMM, Spatz A, Robert C. Cutaneous melanoma. *Lancet.* 2014;383(9919):816–827.

8. Bukowski RM, Tendler C, Cutler D, et al. Treating cancer with PEG intron. *Cancer.* 2002;95(2):389–396.

9. Hansson J, Aamdal S, Bastholt L, et al. Two different durations of adjuvant therapy with intermediate-dose interferon alpha-2b in patients with high-risk melanoma (Nordic IFN trial): a randomised phase 3 trial. *Lancet Oncol.* 2011;12(2):144–152.

10. Eggermont AMM and Gore M. Randomized adjuvant therapy trials in melanoma: surgical and systemic. *Semin Oncol.* 2007;34(6):509–515.

11. Kaufman H, Kim DW, DeRaffele G, et al. Local and distant immunity induced by intralesional vaccination with an oncolytic herpes virus encoding GM-CSF in patients with stage IIIc and IV melanoma. *Ann Surg Oncol.* 2010;17(3):718–730.

12. Eggermont AMM, Chiarion-Sileni V, Grob JJ, et al. Ipilimumab versus placebo after complete resection of stage III melanoma: initial efficacy and safety results from the EORTC 18071 phase III trial. *J Clin Oncol.* 2014;32(15 Suppl):LBA9008.

13. Rosenberg SA, Yang JC, Topalian SL, et al. Treatment of 283 consecutive patients with metastatic melanoma or renal cell cancer using high-dose bolus interleukin 2. *JAMA.* 1994;271(12):907–913.

14. Grimm EA, Mazumder A, Zhang HZ, et al. Lymphokine-activated killer cell phenomenon. Lysis of natural killer-resistant fresh solid tumor cells by interleukin 2-activated autologous human peripheral blood lymphocytes. *J Exper Med.* 1982;155(6):1823–1841.

15. Itoh, K., Platsoucas CD, Balch CM. Autologous tumor-specific cytotoxic T lymphocytes in the infiltrate of human metastatic melanomas. Activation by interleukin 2 and autologous tumor cells, and involvement of the T cell receptor. *J Exper Med.* 1988;168(4):1419–1441.

16. Atkins MB, Lotze MT, Dutcher JP, et al. High-dose recombinant interleukin 2 therapy for patients with metastatic melanoma: analysis of 270 patients treated between 1985 and 1993. *J Clin Oncol.* 1999;17(7):2105.

17. Walker EB, Haley D, Miller W, et al. Gp100(209-2M) peptide immunization of human lymphocyte antigen-A2+ stage I-III melanoma patients induces significant increase in antigen-specific effector and long-term memory CD8+ T cells. *Clin Cancer Res.* 2004;10(2):668–680.

18. Schwartzentruber DJ, Lawson DH, Richards JM, et al. Gp100 peptide vaccine and interleukin-2 in patients with advanced melanoma. *N Engl J Med.* 2011;364(22):2119–2127.

19. Melero I, et al. Immunostimulatory monoclonal antibodies for cancer therapy. *Nat Rev Cancer.* 2007;7(2):95–106.

20. Wolchok JD, Hervas-Stubbs S, Glennie M, et al. Ipilimumab monotherapy in patients with pretreated advanced melanoma: a randomised, double-blind, multicentre, phase 2, dose-ranging study. *Lancet Oncol.* 2010;11(2):155–164.

21. Hodi FS, O'Day SJ, McDermott, DF, et al. Improved survival with ipilimumab in patients with metastatic melanoma. *N Engl J Med.* 2010;363(8):711–723.

22. Okazaki T, Honjo T. PD-1 and PD-1 ligands: from discovery to clinical application. *Int Immunol.* 2007;19(7):813–824.

23. Dong H, Zhu G, Tamada K, et al. B7-H1, a third member of the B7 family, co-stimulates T-cell proliferation and interleukin-10 secretion. *Nat Med.* 1999;5(12):1365–1369.

24. Tseng S-Y, Otsuji M, Gorski K, et al. B7-Dc, a new dendritic cell molecule with potent costimulatory properties for T cells. *J Exper Med.* 2001;193(7):839–846.

25. Zou W, Chen L. Inhibitory B7-family molecules in the tumour microenvironment. *Nat Rev Immunol.* 2008;8(6):467–477.

26. Fife BT, Pauken KE, Eagar TN, et al. Interactions between PD-1 and PD-L1 promote tolerance by blocking the TCR-induced stop signal. *Nat Immunol.* 2009;10(11):1185–1192.

27. Topalian SL, Sznol M, McDermott D, et al. Survival, durable tumor remission, and long-term safety in patients with advanced melanoma receiving nivolumab. *J Clin Oncol.* 2014;32(10):1020–1031.

28. Weber JS, Minor DR, D'Angelo S, et al. A phase 2 randomized, open-labeled study of nivolumab versus investigators' choice chemotherapy (ICC) in patients with advanced melanoma with prior anti-CTLA-4 therapy. Presented at the European Society for Medical Oncology 2014 Congress, Madrid. 2014.

29. Robert C, Ribas A, Wolchok JD, et al. Anti-programmed-death-receptor-1 treatment with pembrolizumab in ipilimumab-refractory advanced melanoma: a randomised dose-comparison cohort of a phase 1 trial. *Lancet.* 2014; 384(9948):1107–1117.

30. Hamid O, Robert C, Daud A, et al. Safety and tumor responses with lambrolizumab (anti–PD-1) in melanoma. *N Engl J Med.* 2013;369(2):134–144.

31. Brahmer JR, Tykodi SS, Chow L, et al. Safety and activity of anti–PD-L1 antibody in patients with advanced cancer. *N Engl J Med.* 2012;366(26):2455–2465.

32. Wolchok JD, Kluger, H, Callahan M, et al. Nivolumab plus ipilimumab in advanced melanoma. *N Engl J Med.* 2013;369(2):122–133.

33. Fu T, He Q, Sharma P. The ICOS/ICOSL pathway is required for optimal antitumor responses mediated by anti–CTLA-4 therapy. *Cancer Res.* 2011;71(16):5445–5454.

34. Topalian SL, Hodi FS, Brahmer JR, et al. Safety, activity, and immune correlates of anti–PD-1 antibody in cancer. *N Engl J Med.* 2012;366(26):2443–2454.

35. Taube JM, Anders RA, Young GD, et al. Colocalization of inflammatory response with B7-H1 expression in human melanocytic lesions

supports an adaptive resistance mechanism of immune escape. *Sci Trans Med.* 2012;4(127):127ra37.

36. Hauschild A, Gogas H, Tarhini A, et al. Practical guidelines for the management of interferon-α-2b side effects in patients receiving adjuvant treatment for melanoma. *Cancer.* 2008;112(5):982–994.

37. Bouwhuis MG, ten Hagen TLM, Eggermont AMM. Immunologic functions as prognostic indicators in melanoma. *Molec Oncol.* 2011;5(2):183–189.

38. Gogas H, Ioannovich J, Dafni U, et al. Prognostic significance of autoimmunity during treatment of melanoma with interferon. *N Engl J Med.* 2006;354(7):709–718.

39. Carella C, Maziotti G, Sorvillo F, et al. Serum thyrotropin receptor antibodies concentrations in patients with Graves' disease before, at the end of methimazole treatment, and after drug withdrawal: evidence that the activity of thyrotropin receptor antibody and/or thyroid response modify during the observation period. *Thyroid.* 2006;16(3):295–302.

40. Weber JS, Kahler KC, Hauschild A. Management of immune-related adverse events and kinetics of response with ipilimumab. *J Clin Oncol.* 2012;30(21):2691–2697.

41. Johnston RL, Lutzky j, Chodhry A, et al. Cytotoxic T-lymphocyte-associated antigen 4 antibody-induced colitis and its management with infliximab. *Dig Dis Sci.* 2009;54(11):2538–2540.

42. Bristol-Myers Squibb: YERVOY (ipilimumab): Serious and fatal immune-mediated adverse reactions—YERVOY risk evaluation and mitigation strategy (REMS). Available at https://www.hcp.yervoy.com/pages/rems.aspx. Published 2012. Accessed July 17, 2015.

Chapter 7

Adjuvant Therapy for High-Risk Melanoma

Radiation Therapy

Michael D. Chuong, Mohammad K. Khan, and Nikhil G. Rao

Overview

While surgical management is the mainstay of treatment for patients with invasive cutaneous melanoma, adjuvant radiation therapy (RT) to the primary site and/or the adjacent nodal regions can provide significant benefit to patients who are at high risk for local or regional recurrence. Due to early preclinical and clinical reports that melanoma is radioresistant, many clinicians have been hesitant to recommend RT.[1] However, subsequent studies have shown melanoma to be responsive to RT, and RT to be a critical component of the comprehensive treatment for select patients with cutaneous melanoma.[2,3] The use of radiotherapy in the future for melanoma is likely to play a greater role, especially combined with newer emerging systemic agents such as CTLA-4 inhibitors, PD-1 inhibitors, BRAF inhibitors, and potential radiation sensitizers such as trametinib.[4–6]

Most cutaneous melanoma patients who are able to undergo adequate local excision of the primary site have a less than 5% risk of local recurrence (LR) and require no additional local therapy.[7] Postoperative RT should be considered, on the other hand, if there is a greater than 10–15% risk of LR. Risk factors for LR include previous LR, positive margins, depth of invasion (Breslow >4 mm), ulceration, satellitosis, perineural infiltration, and angiolymphatic invasion.[7–10]

Desmoplastic Melanoma

A rare melanoma subtype called desmoplastic melanoma (DM) has been reported to inherently have a predisposition for LR. DM accounts for less than 4% of primary cutaneous melanomas and contains melanocytes dispersed in a prominent collagenous stroma with pleomorphic spindle-shaped cells.[10] In addition, DM has a predilection for perineural spread, called *neurotropism*, which results in increased rates of LR.[11] DM tends to be nondescript, amelanotic, and is generally diagnosed at a later stage, often after an initial recurrence, compared with its non-desmoplastic counterpart.[10] As a result, some investigators have advocated the routine use of adjuvant RT to the primary site for DM.

While prospective data are lacking, retrospective studies from the MD Anderson Cancer Center and Moffitt Cancer Center have been reported on DM (Table 7.1). The single-institution study from the Moffitt Cancer Center reviewed a total of 277 patients treated for DM, with 113 receiving adjuvant RT.[12] Both pure (>90% desmoplasia) and mixed subtypes of desmoplastic melanoma were included in the study. Patients who received RT had an improvement in local control, which was particularly noted among patients with positive margins, with tumors involving the head and neck, and with Breslow's thickness greater than 4 mm. Among the 35 patients with positive margins, 14% who received radiation therapy developed LR, versus 54% who did not ($p = 0.004$). This demonstrated the critical importance of consideration of RT in patients with positive margins and other high-risk features. In the series from the MD Anderson Cancer Center, a total of 130 patients were reviewed, and 71 received RT. LR was noted in 24% of the patients who did not receive RT, versus 7% in the group that received RT.[13] Local control was significantly associated with the use of RT ($p = 0.009$).

Stage III Melanoma

Another challenging clinical scenario includes patients who have stage III melanoma with high-risk clinical and pathological features after surgical nodal dissection. Adjuvant RT should be considered in these cases. Increased rates of nodal basin recurrence have been associated with an increasing number of involved nodes (≥3), large nodal size (>3–4 cm), matting of nodes, involvement of cervical nodal basins, and extranodal spread.[14–16] Nodal basin recurrence rates up to 50% have been reported in some patients, many of whom have multiple high-risk features; and there has been a correlation between number of lymph nodes involved melanoma and chance for recurrence.[16–18]

Table 7.1 Retrospective Studies Demonstrating Improved Local Control in Patients Who Received Adjuvant RT for Desmoplastic Melanoma

Moffitt Cancer Center[12]	• 277 total patients; 113 (41%) received adjuvant RT
	• Median follow-up 3.6 years
	• Adjuvant RT reduced local recurrence in patients with positive margin (14% vs. 54%; $P = .004$)
	• Adjuvant RT improved local control ($P < .05$) in patients with negative margins who also had high-risk features (i.e., head and neck location, Breslow depth >4 mm, Clark level V)
MD Anderson Cancer Center[13]	• 130 total patients; 71 (55%) received adjuvant RT
	• Median follow-up 6.6 years
	• Adjuvant RT reduced local recurrence (7% vs. 24%) and was significantly associated with improved local control ($P = .009$) on multivariate analysis

Multiple retrospective series and systematic reviews have suggested that regional control is significantly improved after RT to nodal basins in patients at an increased risk of regional failure.[17,18] In the axilla, the draining basin from the upper extremities or trunk, an increased risk for regional recurrence has been reported after axillary node dissection in patients with extracapsular extension, bulky nodal metastases, and in those with multiple involved lymph nodes.[17] Ballo and colleagues retrospectively reviewed 89 patients with an estimated 30–50% risk of regional recurrence who received a median 30 Gy in five fractions twice weekly over 2.5 weeks. The five-year axillary control and disease-free survival rates were 87% and 46%, respectively, suggesting that RT can effectively limit regional recurrence, although these patients require aggressive systemic therapy to address the risk of distant recurrence.[19] A recent single-institution retrospective study from Australia was published in which the authors aimed to evaluate the anatomical distribution of regionally recurrent disease in patients with stage III melanoma in the axilla, with and without adjuvant RT.[20] A total of 277 patients were treated between 1992 and 2012; 156 did not receive RT, while 121 did receive RT. RT was offered to patients who had two or more involved lymph nodes, an involved lymph node measuring at least 4 cm, or extracapsular extension. RT was prescribed to 48 Gy in 20 fractions and was delivered to the axilla and supraclavicular fossa. Patterns of recurrence differed, based on whether patients received RT. Patients who received RT were more likely to have a recurrence in the adjacent field regions, but were less likely to fail within the treatment field. Regional axillary control after RT was 86%, which is consistent with previously reported series.[19,21,22]

We now have prospective data on the use of radiotherapy in the adjuvant setting for high-risk stage III melanoma. The group from Australia has reported results demonstrating improved regional control after adjuvant RT in patients at high risk for regional failure. Initial data from a phase II trial included 234 patients who received 48 Gy in 20 fractions at a dose of 2.4 Gy per fraction to either the head and neck, axilla and supraclavicular basin, or the illioinguinal basin.[27] Eligible patients had more than one involved node, extracapsular extension, previous regional basin recurrence, or reported intraoperative tumor spill. After in-field recurrences were noted in only 7% of the treated patients, the authors then conducted a randomized trial to further clarify the effect of adjuvant RT in high-risk melanoma patients. Burmeister et al. recently reported results from an international multi-institutional randomized phase III trial that included 123 malignant melanoma patients felt to be at a high risk of nodal relapse following lymphadenectomy.[21] Inclusion criteria included any of one or more of the following: palpable metastatic lymph-node field disease, at least one parotid nodal involvement; at least two cervical or axillary or three involved inguinal nodes; one involved node with extracapsular extension; and one involved node measuring at least 3 cm in greatest diameter in the head and neck or axilla, or 4 cm in the groin. These patients, who were recruited across 16 hospitals in Australia, New Zealand, the Netherlands, and Brazil, were randomized to either observation or adjuvant RT to 48 Gy in 20 fractions. With median follow-up of 40 months, adjuvant RT was found to significantly reduce the risk of lymph node field relapse (hazard ratio [HR] 0.56, 95% confidence interval [CI] 0.32–0.98; $p = .041$) with acceptable early toxicity. However, no differences were detected in either overall survival (HR 1.37, 95% CI 0.94–2.01; $p = .12$) or relapse-free survival (HR 0.91, 95% CI 0.65–1.26; $p = .56$). The primary objective of this study was to show an improvement in local control with the addition of radiotherapy. Randomized patients were selected for very high-risk features ($\geq 25\%$ risk for local recurrence), and as such were also felt to be at very high risk for systemic recurrence. Thus, it is not entirely surprising that there was no statistically significant difference in survival in the two groups of patients. While a previous randomized trial published in 1978 evaluating the role of adjuvant RT was felt to be inconclusive,[28] that study has been criticized for the use of low-energy X-rays, a low total radiation dose, daily fraction size less than 2 Gy, and planned treatment breaks. The importance of the study from Burmeister et al. is that it is the first complete randomized trial within the past several decades to evaluate adjuvant RT with the primary endpoint being lymph node field relapse. Furthermore, it utilized modern RT technique, allowing the results to be evaluated in the context of current-day treatment practices.

Melanoma of the Head and Neck

Melanoma of the head and neck has a propensity for neck nodal metastases and may be associated with a higher rate of recurrence than other nodal basins.[14] This may be due to increased difficulty in achieving widely negative surgical margins. The addition of RT after modified radical or radical neck dissection has consistently been reported to result in regional control rates of up to 90% in clinically node-positive patients (Figure 7.1).[17] However, both surgery and RT can result in significant combined morbidity, including hearing loss, wound breakdown, bone exposure, xerostomia, and ear pain. Moreover, in patients with bilateral nodal metastasis, bilateral cervical radiation has been associated with an unacceptable rate of toxicity and typically is not recommended.[23] Ballo et al. hypothesized that RT may be able to replace formal neck dissection in patients after local excision of nodal disease.[24] Thirty-six patients with parotid or cervical node melanoma metastases had involved nodal excision and omitted a formal neck dissection. Radiation therapy was delivered to the undissected ipsilateral neck, including the site of nodal excision and the primary site. Regional nodal basin recurrences occurred in only two patients, while distant recurrences were detected in 14. The five-year regional control and distant control rates were 93% and 59%. Despite these results, we feel that this approach is not routinely recommended and should only be considered in cases in which patients are unable to undergo completion neck dissection.

A recent publication by Strojan et al. reported their experience using adjuvant RT for melanoma metastases to the neck and/or parotid.[25] A cohort of 43 patients who received adjuvant RT was compared to a cohort of 40 patients who received surgery alone. Negative prognostic factors included three or more involved nodes, at least 3 cm nodal size, extracapsular

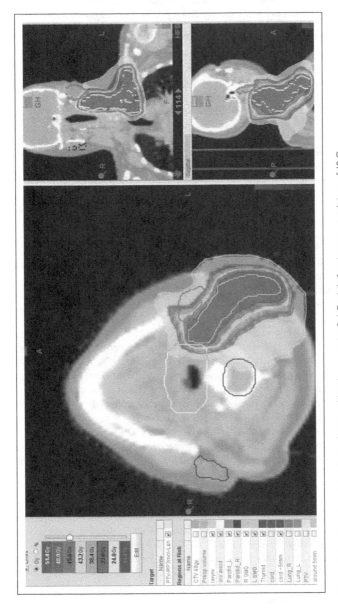

Figure 7.1 Adjuvant neck irradiation for stage III melanoma using 2.4 Gy daily fractions to a total dose of 48 Gy.

extension, close/positive margins, satellitosis, and previous disease recurrence. Two-year regional control was significantly higher in the RT cohort (78% vs. 56%; $p = .015$). Multivariate analysis revealed that RT and the sum of the risk factors present were significant predictors of regional control.

Melanoma of the Lower Extremity

Another nodal basin frequently developing metastatic disease from melanoma of the lower extremities is the inguinal region. Recommendations have been less clear in this anatomical region, given the concerns over toxicity with RT after surgery; particularly, worsening lymphedema and particularly in those with body mass index (BMI) greater than 25–30 kg per meter squared.[17] Recently, there has been a review recommending adjuvant RT to the groin in patients with multiple adverse risk factors, including number of lymph nodes ≥3, size greater than 4 cm, extranodal extension, recurrence and satellitosis. In this series, postoperative RT improved regional control at two years from 46% to 82% ($p = 0.022$) in patients with two or more risk factors.[26] At our center, we are extremely selective in recommending radiation therapy to the inguinal nodal basin and make decisions based on pathological features, postsurgical morbidity, wound healing status, and BMI.

Dose and Fractionation

There are two distinct radiation dose and fractionation strategies for the adjuvant treatment of patients with melanoma. Due to concerns about the relative radioresistance of melanoma cells, investigators initially felt that using a hypofractionated approach with doses per fraction larger than 2 Gy would be most efficacious. The Radiation Therapy Oncology Group (RTOG) has evaluated fraction size for melanoma prospectively in the palliative setting. With the primary endpoint of response at the treated site, 137 patients with measureable metastatic melanoma were randomized to four 8 Gy fractions once weekly over 21 days, versus 20 fractions at 2.5 Gy daily.[29] There was no significant difference in complete response between the arms. However, due to a relatively short follow-up, the toxicity data from this trial are difficult to interpret, and this study is difficult to extrapolate to the postoperative setting.

In the postoperative adjuvant setting, the MD Anderson Cancer Center regimen of 30 Gy in 5 fractions with each fraction separated by at least 72 hours has resulted in excellent disease control.[22,30,31] However, melanoma has also been treated with standard fraction sizes, in part due to concerns about the potential for increased late toxicity with high doses per fraction. When standard fractionation has been used, the total dose has typically been increased to normal tissue tolerance. The University of Florida has reported results using daily 2 Gy fractions to a total of 60 Gy that are similar to those achieved using hypofractionation at 6 Gy per fraction over 2.5 weeks for adjuvant stage III melanoma.[32] The phase III randomized trial by Burmeister et al. delivered fractions at 2.4 gray times 20 daily to a total dose of 48 gray. This may allow some degree of hypofractionation while theoretically limiting the chance for late morbidity.

While there is no consensus on the use of hypofractionated versus standard fractionation RT, it is important to remember that when using hypofractionation, doses above the intended prescription may lead to additional chances for late toxicity and should be minimized. When using the 6 Gy x 5 fraction regimen, the spinal cord, brain, and bowel maximum dose should be kept to less than 24 Gy. Additionally, using modern techniques with 3-D conformal radiation therapy and intensity-modulated radiation therapy may enhance achieving the optimal dose distribution while minimizing irradiation of uninvolved tissues. When using hypofractionation, we are cautious to not treat large volumes of normal tissue and to be cognizant of possible late effects in soft tissue and neural structures.

Lymphedema

After surgical dissection of the axillary nodal basin, patients are at risk to develop lymphedema, and this may be exacerbated by postoperative radiation therapy. In a study by Ballo et al., 26 patients developed treatment-related arm edema after radiation.[19] Classification according to the severity of edema yielded five-year actuarial arm edema rates of 21%, 19%, and 1%, for Grade 1 (transient or asymptomatic), Grade 2 (requiring medical intervention), or Grade 3 (requiring surgical intervention) edema, respectively. Regarding the target volume of radiation therapy in the axilla, Beadle et al. reported their outcomes treating the axilla alone, versus the axilla and the supraclavicular fossa with postoperative radiation therapy at the MD Anderson Cancer Center.[22] The five-year axillary control rate was 88%, with no difference in the two groups. Additionally, there was increased toxicity in the patients who had treatment of the supraclavicular fossa as well. At our center, we do not routinely treat the uninvolved supraclavicular fossa in an attempt to reduce late toxicity including lymphedema and brachial plexopathy.

Conclusion

In summary, prospective and retrospective data demonstrate that melanoma patients with negative clinical and pathological risk factors after resection of the primary lesion and/or regional nodal basin achieve a local and/or regional control benefit from adjuvant RT. Additional studies are needed to clarify the relative risks of individual negative risk factors and specific combinations of risk factors, as well as optimal total dose and fractionation.

References

1. Harwood AR, Cummings BJ. Radiotherapy for malignant melanoma: a re-appraisal. *Cancer treatment reviews*. 1981;8(4):271–282.

2. Stevens G, McKay MJ. Dispelling the myths surrounding radiotherapy for treatment of cutaneous melanoma. *Lancet Oncol*. 2006;7(7):575–583.

3. Rofstad EK. Radiation sensitivity in vitro of primary tumors and metastatic lesions of malignant melanoma. *Cancer Res*. 1992;52(16):4453–4457.

4. Okwan-Duodu D, Pollack BP, Lawson D, Khan MK. Role of radiation therapy as immune activator in the era of modern immunotherapy for metastatic malignant melanoma. *Am J Clin Oncol*. 2015;38(1):119–125.

5. Khan N, Khan MK, Almasan A, Singh AD, Macklis R. The evolving role of radiation therapy in the management of malignant melanoma. *Int J Radiat Oncol Biol Phys*. 2011;80(3):645–654.

6. Khan MK, Khan N, Almasan A, Macklis R. Future of radiation therapy for malignant melanoma in an era of newer, more effective biological agents. *OncoTarg ther*. 2011;4:137–148.

7. Karakousis CP, Balch CM, Urist MM, Ross MM, Smith TJ, Bartolucci AA. Local recurrence in malignant melanoma: long-term results of the multi-institutional randomized surgical trial. *Ann Surg Oncol*. 1996;3(5):446–452.

8. Kelly JW, Sagebiel RW, Calderon W, Murillo L, Dakin RL, Blois MS. The frequency of local recurrence and microsatellites as a guide to reexcision margins for cutaneous malignant melanoma. *Ann Surg*. 1984;200(6):759–763.

9. Urist MM, Balch CM, Soong S, Shaw HM, Milton GW, Maddox WA. The influence of surgical margins and prognostic factors predicting the risk of local recurrence in 3445 patients with primary cutaneous melanoma. *Cancer*. 1985;55(6):1398–1402.

10. Oliver DE, Patel KR, Parker D, et al. The emerging role of radiotherapy for desmoplastic melanoma and implications for future research. *Melanoma Res*. 2015;25(2):95–102. doi: 10.1097/CMR.0000000000000139

11. Chen JY, Hruby G, Scolyer RA, et al. Desmoplastic neurotropic melanoma: a clinicopathologic analysis of 128 cases. *Cancer*. 2008;113(10):2770–2778.

12. Strom T, Caudell JJ, Han D, et al. Radiotherapy influences local control in patients with desmoplastic melanoma. *Cancer*. 2014; 120(9):1369–1378. doi: 10.1002/cncr.28412. Epub 2013 Oct 18

13. Guadagnolo BA, Prieto V, Weber R, Ross MI, Zagars GK. The role of adjuvant radiotherapy in the local management of desmoplastic melanoma. *Cancer*. 2014; 120(9):1361–1368.

14. Bowsher WG, Taylor BA, Hughes LE. Morbidity, mortality and local recurrence following regional node dissection for melanoma. *Br J Surg*. 1986;73(11):906–908.

15. Calabro A, Singletary SE, Balch CM. Patterns of relapse in 1001 consecutive patients with melanoma nodal metastases. *Arch Surg*. 1989;124(9):1051–1055.

16. Lee RJ, Gibbs JF, Proulx GM, Kollmorgen DR, Jia C, Kraybill WG. Nodal basin recurrence following lymph node dissection for melanoma: implications for adjuvant radiotherapy. *Int J Radiat Oncol Biol Phys*. 2000;46(2):467–474.

17. Guadagnolo BA, Zagars GK. Adjuvant radiation therapy for high-risk nodal metastases from cutaneous melanoma. *Lancet Oncol*. 2009;10(4):409–416.

18. Agrawal S, Kane JM 3rd, Guadagnolo BA, Kraybill WG, Ballo MT. The benefits of adjuvant radiation therapy after therapeutic lymphadenectomy for clinically advanced, high-risk, lymph node-metastatic melanoma. *Cancer*. 2009;115(24):5836–5844.

19. Ballo MT, Strom EA, Zagars GK, et al. Adjuvant irradiation for axillary metastases from malignant melanoma. *Int J Radiat Oncol Biol Phys*. 2002;52(4):964–972.

20. Pinkham MB, Foote MC, Burmeister E, et al. Stage III melanoma in the axilla: patterns of regional recurrence after surgery with and without adjuvant radiation therapy. *Int J Radiat Oncol Biol Phys*. 2013;86(4):702–708.

21. Burmeister BH, Henderson MA, Ainslie J, et al. Adjuvant radiotherapy versus observation alone for patients at risk of lymph-node field relapse after therapeutic lymphadenectomy for melanoma: a randomised trial. *Lancet Oncol*. 2012;13(6):589–597.

22. Beadle BM, Guadagnolo BA, Ballo MT, et al. Radiation therapy field extent for adjuvant treatment of axillary metastases from malignant melanoma. *Int J Radiat Oncol Biol Phys.* 2009;73(5):1376–1382.

23. Guadagnolo BA, Myers JN, Zagars GK. Role of postoperative irradiation for patients with bilateral cervical nodal metastases from cutaneous melanoma: a critical assessment. *Head Neck.* 32(6):708–713.

24. Ballo MT, Garden AS, Myers JN, et al. Melanoma metastatic to cervical lymph nodes: Can radiotherapy replace formal dissection after local excision of nodal disease? *Head Neck.* 2005;27(8):718–721.

25. Strojan P, Jancar B, Cemazar M, Perme MP, Hocevar M. Melanoma metastases to the neck nodes: role of adjuvant irradiation. *Int J Radiat Oncol Biol Phys.* 2010;77(4):1039–1045.

26. Gojkovic-Horvat A, Jancar B, Blas M, et al. Adjuvant radiotherapy for palpable melanoma metastases to the groin: When to irradiate? *Int J Radiat Oncol Biol Phys.* 2012;83(1):310–316.

27. Burmeister BH, Smithers BM, Davis S, et al. Radiation therapy following nodal surgery for melanoma: an analysis of late toxicity. *ANZ J Surg.* 2002;72(5):344–348.

28. Creagan ET, Cupps RE, Ivins JC, et al. Adjuvant radiation therapy for regional nodal metastases from malignant melanoma: a randomized, prospective study. *Cancer.* 1978;42(5):2206–2210.

29. Sause WT, Cooper JS, Rush S, et al. Fraction size in external beam radiation therapy in the treatment of melanoma. *Int J Radiat Oncol Biol Phys.* 1991;20(3):429–432.

30. Ballo MT, Ross MI, Cormier JN, et al. Combined-modality therapy for patients with regional nodal metastases from melanoma. *Int J Radiat Oncol Biol Phys.* 2006;64(1):106–113.

31. Stevens G, Thompson JF, Firth I, O'Brien CJ, McCarthy WH, Quinn MJ. Locally advanced melanoma: results of postoperative hypofractionated radiation therapy. *Cancer.* 2000;88(1):88–94.

32. Chang DT, Amdur RJ, Morris CG, Mendenhall WM. Adjuvant radiotherapy for cutaneous melanoma: comparing hypofractionation to conventional fractionation. *Int J Radiat Oncol Biol Phys.* 2006;66(4):1051–1055.

Chapter 8

Follow-up Guidelines for Resected Melanoma

Jeffrey M. Farma and Alia Abdulla

Melanoma is one of the most rapidly growing cancers worldwide, with a consistent increase over the past four decades. There is no consensus for surveillance for patients with resected melanoma. Some studies recommend frequent follow-up visits with abundant use of radiographic imaging and laboratory review, while others question the value of these strategies altogether.[1,2]

According to the National Comprehensive Cancer Network (NCCN), the lifetime risk of developing a second primary melanoma approaches 4–8%, therefore lifetime dermatological surveillance is recommended.[3] However, longitudinal care varies worldwide, and guidelines are disparate. Lifelong follow-up is important because of the risk of (1) second primary melanomas, (2) locoregional recurrence, (3) late recurrence, and (4) other cutaneous malignancies. Risk of local recurrence is greatest in the first five years after diagnosis, especially in thick and ulcerated tumors.[4] Locoregional recurrence of melanoma is defined as recurrence at the site of the primary lesion, regionally in the draining lymph node basin, or in between. Satellite and in-transit metastases are distinguished by their distance from the primary site, with satellite lesions occurring within 2 cm and in-transit metastases occurring more than 2 cm from the primary lesion (Figure 8.1). Both satellite and in-transit metastases are considered stage IIIB (without regional nodal metastases) or stage IIIC (with regional nodal metastases) disease (American Joint Committee on Cancer, 7th ed.).[3]

Dermatological Surveillance

Dermatological surveillance includes total-body skin examination, palpation of the primary site and surrounding area for local recurrences or in-transit metastases, and a thorough regional lymph node basin examination. Review of systems should be specific and include questions about new or changing lesions, weight loss, fatigue, headache, new back pain, and any new symptoms that have persisted. Patients should be counseled to adhere to sun-protective measures and perform skin self-examinations.

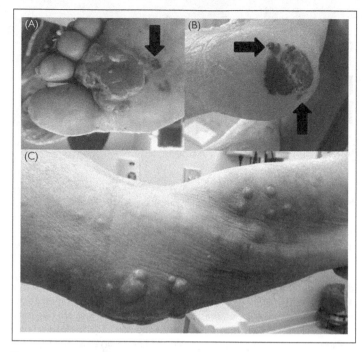

Figure 8.1 *A*, Plantar aspect of the foot with melanoma and satellite lesions (arrow). *B*, Heel with melanoma surrounded by satellite lesions (arrows). *C*, In-transit nodules of the upper extremity with a primary distal upper extremity melanoma.

Total Cutaneous Examination

Regular skin surveillance with monthly self-examination and total cutaneous examination (TCE) by a dermatologist increases the chances of detecting thinner melanomas, reducing morbidity and mortality. However, there are no controlled trials evaluating TCE on melanoma mortality. Berwick et al. describe a link between regular skin self-examination and reduction in the risk of developing advanced melanoma, reducing melanoma mortality by 63%.[5] De Giorgi et al. evaluated 802 patients retrospectively and found that 36% of melanomas were discovered during annual skin examinations by dermatologists and 33% were discovered by patients. Further analysis revealed that self-detection was associated with a greater probability of having a thicker melanoma.[6]

A follow-up protocol at the Yale Melanoma Unit in 1987 aimed at improving the detection of recurrence in patients with stage I to III melanoma. The protocol consisted of a patient-education program and a standardized follow-up schedule. A retrospective evaluation of 419 patients treated from January 1988 to December 1994 revealed that among 78 patients with disease recurrence, 34 (44%) had clinical symptoms, raising suspicion of metastases that were initially detected by the patients. Fifty-six percent of recurrences were detected by physician-directed surveillance examinations.[7] Most recurrences were found within the first (47%) or second (32%) year of follow-up. The study recommended surveillance schedules as follows: (1) stage I, annually; (2) stage II, every six months for years 1–2 and annually thereafter; (3) stage III, every three months for year 1, every four months for year 2, and every six months for years 3–5; (4) at year 6 and beyond, all patients should have surveillance annually, due to the risk of late recurrence and/or multiple primaries.[7]

Garbe et al. prospectively analyzed 2008 patients within a single institution in Germany. Two hundred thirty-three metastatic recurrences and 62 second or multiple primary melanomas were discovered during the 25-month study period. More than 70% of recurrences were detected on scheduled follow-up examinations, and 17% of all recurrences were first discovered by the patients. Physical examination diagnosed 50% of recurrences; the remaining 50% were detected radiographically.[8] The Scottish Melanoma Group found that almost half (47%) of recurrences were first observed by the patient, with only 26% being initially detected on follow up.[9] Garbe et al. classified recurrences as "early" or "late" phase of development, and patients diagnosed in the early phase had significantly more favorable odds of recurrence-free and overall survival than those in a late phase. They recommended examination by TCE every six months for five years in stage I with ≤1 mm thickness, every three months for five years in stage I and II with >1 mm thickness, and every three months for first three years for stage III. For years 6–10, the physical examination can be spaced such that it is every 12 months in stage I with ≤1 mm thickness, every six months in stage I and II with >1 mm thickness, and every six months for stage III.[8]

According to the NCCN, the recommended follow-up for stage 0 is annually, for stage IA to IIA is every 6–12 months for first five years, and for stage IIB to IV is every 3–6 months for the first two years, then every 3–12 months for the next three years, then annually.[3] The American Academy of Dermatology (AAD) published guidelines for follow-up of resected melanoma in November 2011 stating that no clear data regarding follow-up intervals exist, and at least annual examinations with interval self-examinations are necessary.[10] Table 8.1 summarizes the major recommendations for follow-up examinations currently published.

Total Cutaneous Photography

Total cutaneous photography (TCP) was initially described in 1988 by William Slue as a method of taking total-body photographs to document dysplastic nevi. Photos are used for comparison at subsequent follow-up examinations. Detection of thin malignant melanomas in a curable stage is enhanced by utilizing these baseline photographs.[15] Currently, TCP has evolved into a system involving digital photography-based mole mapping. Patients who are high risk with multiple nevi can use the photographs to assist in self-examinations. Feit et al. reported an increase in the melanoma diagnosis rate with the use of this technique. Moreover, they reported that melanomas identified with the assistance of TCP are generally thin melanomas.[16] However, there are barriers to the increased use of TCP, including the cost, which tends not to be covered

Table 8.1 Surveillance Examination Guidelines for Resected Melanoma

	Surveillance Physical Examination						
	Stage 0	Stage IA	Stage IB	Stage IIA	Stage IIB	Stage III	Stage IV
NCCN[3]	Annually	Every 6–12 mo, Yrs 1–5, then as clinically indicated			Every 6–12 mo, Yrs 1–2 Every 3–12 mo, Yrs 3–5, then annually		
AAD[10]	At least annual examinations						
GMG[8,11]			Every 6 mo, Yrs 1–3 Every 12 mo, Yrs 4–5, then annually		Every 3 mo, Yrs 1–3 Every 3–6 mo, Yrs 4–5 Every 6 mo, Yrs 5–10		
UK[12]			Every 3 mo, Yrs 1–3, then no further follow-up		Every 3 mo, Yrs 1–3 Every 6 mo, Yrs 4–5		
ESMO[13]	No consensus						
CCA[14]			Every 6 mo, Yrs 1–5, then annually		Every 3–4 mo, Yrs 1–5, then annually		
YMU[7]			Annually	Every 6 mo, Yrs 1–2, then annually		Every 3 mo, Yr 1 Every 4 mo, Yr 2 Every 6 mo, Yr 3–5, then annually	
SMG[9]			Every 3 mo, Yrs 1–3, then annually Yrs 4–5, nothing after Yr 5				

NCCN: National Comprehensive Cancer Network; AAD: American Academy of Dermatology; GMG: German Melanoma Guidelines; UK: UK Guidelines; ESMO: European Society for Medical Oncology; CCA: Cancer Council Australia; YMU: Yale Melanoma Unit; SMG: Scottish Melanoma Group.

by insurance; having the photos available during physical examinations; and a medico-legal concern about the potential of these photographs to be used in malpractice suits.[17]

Laboratory Tests

Currently, there are two potential tumor markers for melanoma, including lactate dehydrogenase (LDH) and S100β. LDH is found throughout the body, and is expressed by a multitude of cancers and non-malignant etiologies; however, it is unsuitable for use in screening or diagnosis of melanoma. Persistent or recurrent elevations of LDH after treatment of melanoma may indicate residual or recurrent disease. Another novel marker is serum protein S100β, which was first described in 1980 in cultured melanoma cells and is an immunohistochemical marker of pigmented skin lesions.

Finck et al. reported 121 stage II and 58 stage III patients in whom high levels of LDH indicated recurrence with a sensitivity and specificity of 72% and 97%, respectively. As an indicator of liver metastasis, LDH had a sensitivity and specificity of 95% and 82%, respectively, in stage II melanoma; and 86%

and 57%, respectively, in stage III melanoma. An elevated LDH was the first indication of recurrent disease in 11 of 88 (12.5%) stage II patients. The mean survival following LDH elevation was 5.9 months. It was concluded that monitoring LDH can provide useful information in the postoperative follow-up of patients with melanoma.[18] Other reports have documented an association between serum levels of LDH and prognosis in patients with stage IV melanoma; however, the prognostic value of LDH in patients with stage I–III melanoma is very limited, as it is rarely elevated.

In a retrospective analysis of 261 patients with a regimented follow-up schedule, 145 evaluable patients developed recurrent melanomas. Ninety-nine patients (68%) developed clinical symptoms that initiated a workup for recurrence. Physical examination of asymptomatic patients led to the diagnosis of recurrent disease in 37 patients (26%). The other nine patients (6%) with recurrent disease had abnormal chest X-rays (CXR). Laboratory results were never a sole indicator of recurrent disease. They concluded that blood analyses and CXR have limited value in the follow-up of patients with resected intermediate- and high-risk melanomas.[19]

Garbe et al. evaluated 1,492 patients on whom 2,719 blood tests (including blood count, erythrocyte sedimentation rate, renal function, liver enzymes, LDH, and S100β) were performed annually in the earlier stages, and twice yearly in patients with more advanced-stage melanoma. Blood tests were rarely the first sign of metastasis, and a diagnosis was made in only three patients after the detection of an elevated LDH. In patients developing metastasis, LDH and alkaline phosphatase (AP) were found to be elevated in 16.4% and 12.5%, respectively. Both percentages were significantly higher than in patients without metastasis (4.2% for LDH and 3.5% for AP, $P < .0001$). Half of these patients with stage II and III disease expressed serum protein S100β, and it was elevated in approximately 50% of patients with distant metastasis. In patients with locoregional recurrence, only a few were found to have an elevated protein S100β.[8]

Routine blood tests contribute to the detection of metastasis in a very small subset of patients. Nevertheless, increasing values of both markers, LDH and serum protein S100β, may be the first sign of recurrence. Future investigations are needed to clarify whether protein S100β is a suitable substitute for the other blood values or whether it should be used as a supplementary examination method. Currently, the use of laboratory tests in the surveillance of earlier stage melanoma is not recommended (see Table 8.2).

Imaging

Currently, there are no formal imaging guidelines for surveillance in patients with resected melanomas. According to the NCCN, additional radiological imaging is only recommended based on symptoms.[3] CXR, computed tomography (CT), and/or positron emission tomography/CT (PET/CT) are considered optional and should be tailored to the stage and the discretion of the physician.[3] Guidelines recommend "considering" radiological studies every 4–12 months in stage IIB or greater.[3] Published guidelines for the management

Table 8.2 Surveillance Laboratory Tests and Imaging Guidelines for Resected Melanoma

	Laboratory Studies		Radiological Studies		
	LDH	S100β	LNUS	CXR	PET/CT
NCCN[3]	NR	NR	Consider*	Consider every 4–12 mo ≥ stage IIB	
AAD[10]	NR	NR	NR	NR	NR
GMG[8,11]	**	Every 3mo ≥ stage 1B for Yrs 1–3, every 6 mo, thereafter Yrs 4–5 if ≥ stage IIC	Every 6 mo, stage IB–IIB / Every 3 mo, ≥ stage IIC	NR	Every 6 mo, ≥ stage IIC for Yrs 1–3
UK[12]	**	**	NR	NR	NR
ESMO[13]	No consensus				
CCA[14]	**	**	Advanced disease	**	**

LNUS: Lymph node ultrasonography; NCCN: National Comprehensive Cancer Network; AAD: American Academy of Dermatology; GMG: German Melanoma Guidelines; UK: UK Guidelines; ESMO: European Society for Medical Oncology; CCA: Cancer Council Australia; NR: not recommended.

*Consider only if equivocal lymph node physical examination, patients were offered but did not undergo sentinel lymph node biopsy, or patients with a positive sentinel lymph node biopsy who did not undergo complete lymph node dissection.
**No recommendation.

of cutaneous melanoma in the United Kingdom, the Netherlands, and Australia do not recommend routine radiological investigations; however, German guidelines recommend cross-sectional imaging every six months for stage IIC or greater for the first three years after resection. Swiss guidelines recommend annual CXRs for the first five years in patients with stage I/II disease, and PET/CT or CT in the follow-up of stage III patients.[11,20] Table 8.2 summarizes radiology recommendations for patients with melanoma.

Chest X-ray

A common site of distant spread for melanoma is to the lungs. Surveillance CXRs have a high number of false-positive and false-negative findings. Morton et al. studied the accuracy of surveillance CXRs and the impact on survival by evaluating extent of distant disease, time to detection, and treatment in those with CXR-detected compared with symptomatic pulmonary metastases. One hundred and eight high-risk patients were followed with CXR every six months for eight years and then annually until 10 years. 21% (23/108) of the high-risk patients developed pulmonary metastases, but only 10% were detected by CXR. Sensitivity and specificity of surveillance CXRs were 48% and 78%, respectively, with a high false-positive rate. Only 13% (3/23) of the identified pulmonary metastases were amenable to surgical intervention.[20] Leiter et al. showed a benefit in use of chest X-ray only in stage III disease. This study prospectively followed 1,969 patients, and only 10/204 relapses were discovered by chest X-ray. The majority (7/10) of recurrences were in patients with stage III disease.[21] Brown et al. reported a low sensitivity of 7.7%

and a specificity of 96.5%. In a trial of 1,235 patients, 210 relapses occurred, 38 of which were detected by CXR. In order to detect these 38 recurrences, a total of 4,218 (38/4218 = 0.9%) X-rays were performed, with a 129 (3.1%) false-positive rate. Isolated pulmonary metastases amenable to resection were found in only 3 of 38 patients.[22]

In conclusion, CXR does not dependably identify pulmonary metastases, nor has it led to earlier detection of pulmonary metastases. In most series, when pulmonary metastases are detected, they are generally unresectable. Frequent CXR surveillance can cause unnecessary patient anxiety, given high false-positive rates, as well as incurring significant medical costs.

Lymph Node Ultrasonography

Lymph node ultrasonography is noninvasive, takes little time, and is cost-effective. Ultrasonography examines the surgical scar of the primary tumor, the in-transit area, the locoregional lymph nodes, and potentially further lymph node basins. Lymph node ultrasonography has been described as an effective procedure for the early detection of locoregional lymph node metastases.[21,23] Ulrich et al. demonstrated lymph node ultrasonography to be superior in detecting metastases, with a sensitivity and specificity of 99.2% and 98.3%, respectively, as opposed to 25.2% and 98.4% with physical examination.[24] Garbe et al. had similar results supporting ultrasound and reported 71% early detection compared to 48% early detection for all examination methods[8]; however, there is an associated higher rate of false positives (1.6%) compared to physical examination (0.66%).[21] In contrast to these studies, Chai et al. evaluated lymph node ultrasonography's ability to identify a concordant result on sentinel lymph node biopsy by performing ultrasound in the preoperative setting. Overall the sensitivity was 33.8%, specificity 85.7%, positive predictive value 36.5%, and negative predictive value 84.2%.[25] Therefore lymph node ultrasonography has shown neither a consistently high sensitivity nor specificity for diagnosis of nodal metastases. However, its utility can still be of benefit in some settings, especially when sentinel lymph node biopsies or completion lymph node dissections (when indicated) are not performed due to other factors (comorbidities, sentinel lymph node failed to map, or refusal by patient).

Neither the NCCN nor the AAD include this technique in their recommendations.[3,10] The NCCN states that lymph node ultrasound may be considered in patients with an equivocal physical examination, in patients who were offered sentinel lymph node biopsy but refused, or patients with positive sentinel lymph nodes who did not receive complete lymph node dissections.[3] German melanoma guidelines, however, do recommend lymph node ultrasonography every six months in stage IB to IIB and every three months for stage IIC or greater.[11]

Computed Tomography and Magnetic Resonance Imaging

Magnetic resonance imaging (MRI) can more readily detect cerebral metastases than can CT and PET/CT.[26] MRI has proven to be more sensitive and specific in the detection of soft-tissue and osseous metastases as well,[27] but there are no strong data directly comparing MRI to CT in osseous metastasis.[28]

Whole-body CT is a sensitive procedure, which allows for the detection of metastases as small as 2–4 mm.[27] In a study by Romano et al., 72% of asymptomatic distant metastases were discovered by CT scans,[1] while other trials yielded detection rates of 15–28%.[8] During follow-up of patients with stage IV disease and in cases of suspected metastasis, CT plays a pivotal role. More than 50% of recurrences in asymptomatic stage III patients are detected by the patient or by examinations; thus cross-sectional imaging screening should only be performed in high-risk patients.[1,8,29] CT has a higher sensitivity compared to MRI in the diagnosis of small pulmonary metastases (66.9 vs. 2.9%, $p < 0.0001$) and should be considered.[27] Drawbacks to CT are its limited soft-tissue contrast, cost, and radiation exposure.

Positron Emission Tomography/Computed Tomography

PET/CT displays the uptake of radioactively labeled glucose in metabolically active areas. In a meta-analysis evaluating imaging modalities in surveillance of melanoma patients, PET/CT revealed a high sensitivity (80%) and specificity (87%) in the detection of distant metastases, higher than conventional CT (51% and 69%, respectively).[23] Rinne et al. studied 100 patients prospectively and found an increase in sensitivity from 20% to 71.4% when comparing conventional diagnostic techniques to PET/CT.[26] The NCCN recommends considering PET/CT every 4–12 months in stage IIB or higher-stage melanoma patients.[3] According to the AAD, surveillance imaging studies in asymptomatic patients have low yield for detection of metastases and are associated with high false-positive rates.[10] Overall, a general recommendation on imaging procedures cannot be made based on current data, as the studies included inhomogeneous patients groups and are characterized by low evidence levels (see Table 8.2).

Conclusion

The major benefit of dermatological surveillance is to detect potentially curable recurrence, especially resectable locoregional recurrences. Surveillance laboratory tests and CXRs can have limited value while producing a relatively high false-positive rate. Lymph node ultrasonography is a valuable imaging modality in patients with equivocal lymphatic nodal basin physical examinations. In patients with early stages of melanoma, the benefit of routine surveillance imaging studies is questionable, and we do not generally perform this at our institution; however, close surveillance with detailed medical history and physical examination is necessary, with special attention to regional recurrences every three to 12 months, depending on the AJCC stage category the patient falls into and the risk of recurrence. In stage III or greater, more frequent surveillance in the form of more frequent physical examination, laboratory tests based on symptomatology, and cross-sectional imaging may be indicated because of the higher risk of recurrence in this population. CT, MRI, and PET/CT are often a component of the overall follow-up for these high-risk patients. Additional studies are needed to better define the role of surveillance in the asymptomatic patient with resected melanoma.

References

1. Romano E, Scordo M, Dusza SW, Coit DG, Chapman PB. Site and timing of first relapse in stage III melanoma patients: implications for follow-up guidelines. *J Clin Oncol.* 2010;28(18):3042–3047.

2. Crowley NJ, Seigler HF. Late recurrence of malignant melanoma. *Ann Surg* 1990;212(2):173–177.

3. NCCN. National Comprehensive Cancer Network Clinical Practice Guidelines in Oncology—v.2.2014: Melanoma. Available at http://www.nccn.org/professionals/physician_gls/pdf/melanoma.pdf. Accessed September 30, 2013.

4. Bolognia JL, Jorizzo JL, Schaffer JV. *Dermatology*, 3rd ed. Elsevier Limited: Saunders, 2012:1905–1910.

5. Berwick M, Begg CB, Fine JA, Roush GC, Barnhill RL. Screening for cutaneous melanoma by skin self-examination. *J Natl Cancer Inst.* 1996;88(1):17–23.

6. De Giorgi V, Grazzini M, Rossari S, et al. Is skin self-examination for cutaneous melanoma detection still adequate? A retrospective study. *Dermatology.* 2012;225(1):31–36.

7. Poo-Hwu WJ, Ariyan S, Lamb L, et al. Follow-up recommendations for patients with American Joint Committee on Cancer stages I–III malignant melanoma. *Cancer.* 1999;86(11):2252–2258.

8. Garbe C, Paul A, Kohler-Spath H, et al. Prospective evaluation of a follow-up schedule in cutaneous melanoma patients: recommendations for an effective follow-up strategy. *J Clin Oncol.* 2003;21(3):520–529.

9. Dicker TJ, Kavanagh GM, Herd RM, et al. A rational approach to melanoma follow-up in patients with primary cutaneous melanoma. *Br J Dermatol.* 1999;140(2):249–254.

10. Bichakjian CK, Halpern AC, Johnson TM, et al. Guidelines of care for the management of primary cutaneous melanoma. *J Am Acad Dermatol.* 2011;65(5):1032–1047.

11. Pflugfelder A, Kochs C, Blum A, et al. Malignant melanoma S3-Guideline: "Diagnosis, therapy and follow-up of melanoma." *J Dtsch Dermatol Ges.* 2013;11(6):1–116.

12. Roberts DL, Anstey AV, Barlow RJ, et al. U.K. guidelines for the management of cutaneous melanoma. *Br J Dermatol.* 2002;146:7–17.

13. Dummer R, Hauschild A, Guggenheim M, Keilholz U, Pentheroudakis G. Cutaneous melanoma: ESMO Clinical Practice Guidelines for diagnosis, treatment, and follow-up. *Ann Oncol.* 2012;23(7):vii86–vii91.

14. Clinical Practice Guidelines for the Management of Melanoma in Australia and New Zealand. Available at www.nhmrc.gov.au/guidelines/publications/cp111. Accessed Sept. 30, 2013.

15. Slue W, Kopf AW, Rivers JK. Total-body photographs of dysplastic nevi. *Arch Dermatol.* 1988;124(8):1239–1243.

16. Feit NE, Dusza SW, Marghoob AA. Melanomas detected with the aid of total cutaneous photograph. *Br J Dermatol.* 2004;150(4):706–714.

17. Halpern AC. The use of whole body photography in a pigmented lesion clinic. *Dermatol Surg.* 2000;26(12):1175–1180.

18. Finck SJ, Giuliano AE, Morton DL. LDH and melanoma. *Cancer.* 1983;51(5):840–843.

19. Weiss M, Loprinzi CL, Creagan ET, Dalton RJ, Novotny P, O'Fallon JR. Utility of follow-up tests for detecting recurrent disease in patients with malignant melanomas. *JAMA*. 1995;274(21):1703–1705.

20. Morton RL, Craig JC, Thompson JF. The role of surveillance chest X-rays in the follow-up of high-risk melanoma patients. *Ann Surg Oncol*. 2009;16(3):571–577.

21. Leiter U, Marghoob AA, Lasithiotakis K. Costs of the detection of metastases and follow-up examinations in cutaneous melanoma. *Melanoma Res*. 2009;19(1):50–57.

22. Brown RE, Stromberg AJ, Hagendoorn LJ, et al. Surveillance after surgical treatment of melanoma: futility of routine chest radiography. *Surgery*. 2010;148(4):711–716.

23. Xing Y, Bronstein Y, Ross, et al. Contemporary diagnostic imaging modalities for the staging and surveillance of melanoma patients: a meta-analysis. *J Natl Cancer Inst*. 2011;103(2):129–142.

24. Ulrich J, van Akkooi AJC, Eggermont AMM, Voit C. New developments in melanoma: utility of ultrasound imaging (initial staging, follow-up and pre-SLNB). *Expert Rev Anticancer Ther*. 2011;11(11):1693–1701.

25. Chai C, Zager J, Szabunio M, et al. Preoperative ultrasound is not useful for identifying nodal metastasis in melanoma patients undergoing sentinel node biopsy: preoperative ultrasound in clinically node-negative melanoma. *Ann Surg Oncol*. 2012;19:1100–1106.

26. Rinne D, Baum RP, Hor G, Kaufmann R. Primary staging and follow-up of high risk melanoma patients with whole-body ^{18}F-fluorodeoxyglucaose positron emission tomography. *Cancer*. 1998;82(9):1664–1671.

27. Hausmann D, Jochum S, Utikal J, et al. Comparison of the diagnostic accuracy of whole-body MRI and whole-body CT in stage III/IV malignant melanoma. *J Dtsch Dermatol Ges*. 2011;9(3):212–222.

28. Pfannenberg C, Aschoff P, Schanz S, et al. Prospective comparison of ^{18}F-fluorodeoxyglucose positron emission tomography/computed tomography and whole-body magnetic resonance imaging in staging of advanced malignant melanoma. *Eur J Cancer*. 2007;43(3):557–564.

29. Francken AB, Bastiaannet E, Hoekstra HJ. Follow-up in patients with localised primary cutaneous melanoma. *Lancet Oncol*. 2005;6(8):608–621.

Chapter 9

Metastatic Melanoma

Targeted Therapy

Kathryn Baksh and Ragini R. Kudchadkar

Melanoma Biology

Transformation into melanoma is thought to occur due to the accumulation of mutations in growth-regulating genes, the loss of adhesion receptors, and the increase in autocrine and paracrine growth factors; all of which contribute to uncontrolled proliferation promoting the survival of these abnormal cells.[1] The response rates of melanoma to traditional cytotoxic agents have been in the range of 6–15%.[2] In addition, chemotherapy alone has not been able to proven to improve overall survival for patients with this disease. These circumstances set the stage for the exploration into the melanoma genome and the development of novel targeted agents to manipulate the respective molecular pathways.

Over the last decade, targeted therapies based on the molecular aberrancies in melanoma have revolutionized the treatment of this disease. The identification of genetic abnormalities leading to aberrant signal transduction in melanoma cells has been the basis of targeted drug development in melanoma. The mutation rate of melanoma exceeds those of other malignancies, and this is thought to be related to ultraviolet radiation exposure link to melanoma development.[3] One pathway of particular interest is the mitogen-activated protein kinase (MAPK) pathway. The MAPK pathway consists of a cascade of three kinases, the rapidly accelerated fibroblast (RAF) family of kinases, the MAPK/extracellular-signal-regulated kinase (MEK1/2), and terminating with the extracellular signal-regulated kinase (ERK). Once activated through RAF and MEK, ERK can then migrate to the nucleus to drive cell proliferation through the activation of cyclin D1 and down-regulation of p27. Under normal cell signaling, activation of this pathway occurs through ligand binding to a transmembrane receptor. However, mutations can lead to aberrant protein signaling that causes this pathway to be constitutively active. Increased MAPK signaling is an early event that is required, but not sufficient alone, to cause melanoma; i.e., multiple events are required, including the activation of the MAPK pathway, to lead to the development of melanoma.[1,4,5,6]

Various mutations have been identified to drive the MAPK pathway in melanoma. Approximately 20% patients with melanoma have *NRAS* mutations;

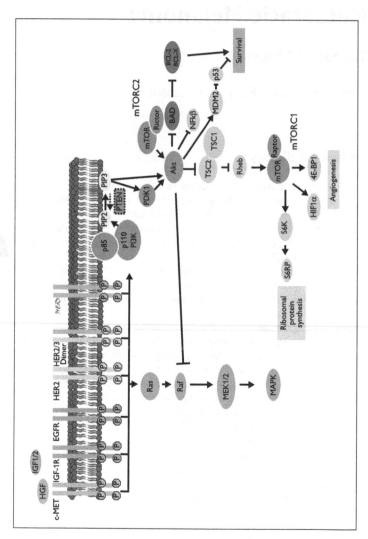

Figure 9.1 MAPK pathway. Modified and reprinted with permission from Yap TA et al. *J Clin Oncol.* 2013;31:1592–1605.

Table 9.1 Melanoma Types and Most Commonly Associated Mutations	
Types of Melanoma	**Most Common Mutations**
Cutaneous Melanoma	*BRAF, NRAS*
– Superficial Spreading Melanoma	
– Nodular Melanoma	
Mucosal Melanoma	*KIT, NRAS, BRAF*
Acral Lentiginous Melanoma	*KIT*
Ocular Melanoma	*GNAQ, GNA11*

50–60% harbor a mutation in *BRAF. KIT* alterations are seen very rarely (1%) overall in all types of melanoma, but are seen in 10–15% of acral or mucosal melanomas. At least half of uveal melanomas harbor a distant mutation, *GNAQ/GNA11*.[7,8,9] All these mutational changes lead to increased signaling through the MAPK pathway (Figure 9.1), thus causing increases in the proteins MEK and ultimately ERK that signal into the nucleus of the cell in order to drive proliferation (see Table 9.1).

In addition to increased signaling through the MAPK pathway, up-regulation of the phosphoinositide 3-kinase (PI3K) pathway has also been identified. The PI3K pathway has been found to be activated in melanoma by activating mutations in the signaling molecules, deletion of the phosphatase and tensin homology (PTEN) or overexpression/activation of receptor tyrosine kinases. Distant mutation in genes involved in this pathway is not as clear as it has been in MAPK signaling alterations. These alterations are not only involved in the biology of melanoma but are also key factors in resistance to *BRAF* inhibitors.[10,11,12]

In the rest of the chapter, we will discuss how current therapies for metastatic melanoma manipulate these biological alternations in melanoma and lead to improved outcomes for patients with this disease.

Single-Agent *BRAF* Inhibition Vemurafenib and Dabrafenib

As discussed previously, 50–60% of melanomas carry an activating mutation of *BRAF*.[13,14] The vast majority (approximately 80%) of *BRAF* mutations result from substitution of glutamic acid for valine at amino acid 600 (V600E).[8] *BRAF* mutations tend to be more common on body sites that are intermittently exposed to the sun. *BRAF* mutational status correlates with the age of the patient, with younger patients having an increased incidence of melanoma.[15,16] The other approximately 15% of *BRAF* mutations results in a substituted lysine for valine (*BRAF* V600K). Rarer *BRAF* mutations do exist. The most common alternatives to V600E and K are V600D,R which susbstitue valine to aspartic acid or arginine respectively in the *BRAF* gene. These alternative mutations are seen more frequently in older patients and are thought to arise in individuals with a high amount of accumulated sun damage.[17]

In the United States, the Food and Drug Administration (FDA) has approved two single-agent drugs to effectively block the *BRAF* protein. These *BRAF* inhibitors, vemurafenib (Zelobraf®) and dabrafenib (Tafinlar®), have been shown to improve overall survival over chemotherapy in patients with unresectable stage III and IV melanoma. Vemurafenib clinical trials have shown an approximately 50% response rate [RR] (indicating a greater than 30% reduction in tumor burden), with an additional 20–30% of patients experiencing stability of the disease.[18,19,20] BRIM-2 (*BRAF* In Melanoma) was a phase II trial evaluating vemurafenib at 960 mg by mouth, twice daily (PO BID) in the treatment-refractory metastatic melanoma population, and demonstrated a median survival of 15.9 months in the 132 patients treated.[20] Median overall survival using single-agent BRIM-3 was the phase III registration trial that led to this drug's approval. In this study, 675 patients were randomized to dacarbazine or vemurafenib. The six-month overall survival rates were 84% and 64%, respectively.[19] Due to the significant benefit, the study was closed in January 2011 to allow crossover to the vemurafenib arm. In August of 2011, the FDA approved vemurafenib for the treatment of *BRAF* V600E mutated metastatic melanoma in the treatment-naïve or refractory settings.

In May of 2013, a second *BRAF* inhibitor, dabrafenib (150 mg PO BID), was approved by the FDA secondary to overall survival benefit over dacarbazine. The phase III study of this agent established a 50% RR to the agent and an improved progression-free survival [PFS] of 5.1 months versus 2.7 months over dacarbazine.[21]

Both *BRAF* inhibitors were compared to dacarbazine, as this was the only approved agent and had been the standard of care for patients with stage IV melanoma at the time of initiation of these trials. Ipilimumab was approved in 2011, but was not available at the time of these studies. BRAF inhibitors have yet to be studied head to head with immunotherapy, though many combination studies are ongoing. The most appropriate sequencing of immunotherapy and *BRAF* inhibitors has yet to be established by a randomized, prospective study. However, many experts believe that immunotherapy should be offered first if clinically appropriate, as it offers more durable responses, and retrospective data indicate that immunotherapy may not be as effective after treatment with a *BRAF* inhibitor.[22] Retrospective data though is clearly biased as patients starte on targeted therapy upfront may have had biologically and clinically more aggressive disease as this is the population that is typically started on immunotherapy upfront. A trial via a Eastern Oncology Cooperative Group just started in enrollment that will randomize patients to receive either immunotherapy or targeted therapy upfront with cross over at progression.

Vemurafenib and dabrafenib do differ slightly, though both inhibit the mutated *BRAF* protein. Studies with dabrafenib included both V600E- and K-mutated melanoma, whereas vemurafenib studies only included V600E-mutated melanoma. Response rates are similar in both populations, though slightly higher for the V600E mutated group. Ongoing studies are evaluating vemurafenib in the non-E-mutated population (NCT01586195). Dabrafenib has a shorter-half compared to vemurafenib and has slightly different side-effect profile. Pyrexia is much more common with dabrafenib, and skin toxicities are more common with vemurafenib, though both the skin toxicities and fevers can potentially occur with either agent.

The most common toxicities noted on trials are fatigue, arthralgias, fevers, hand-foot syndrome, and non-melanoma skin cancers, specifically well-differentiated squamous cell carcinomas.[18–21] The cutaneous side effects are believed to arise from the induction of hypoproliferative phenotypes by these agents. These phenotypes result in keratodermas, keratosis pilaris, papillomas, keratoacanthomas, and squamous cell carcinomas. The hypoproliferative effects are believed to occur secondary to paradoxical activation of the pathway in which the BRAF inhibitor promotes MEK activation in normal cells that have activation of upstream receptors or signaling molecules.[23] It is always a concern when an anti-neoplastic agent promotes the proliferation of neoplastic lesions. Long-term safety studies are needed on patients being treated with these agents.

Dose reductions in vemurafenib or dabrafenib are effective in decreasing the side-effect profiles of these agents. Low-dose steroids (e.g., prednisone 10 mg daily) chronically are effective to maintain patients on these agents and decrease symptoms of fevers, arthralgias, hand-foot syndrome, and rash. For more severe rashes, a slow steroid taper and drug hold is effective as well. Rapid reductions in steroids as seen in a traditional methylprednisolone dosepak can lead to increased flares of dermatitis. Vemurafenib can be dose-reduced to as low as 480 mg PO BID, and dabrafenib to 75 mg PO BID. Below these doses, effective BRAF inhibition does not occur.

The high response rates seen with these agents had not been seen in melanoma before, leading to much hope for the promise of these agents. However, the median time to progression is approximately six months, indicating that acquired resistance of melanoma to these agents develops relatively quickly. Research shows that about 50% of patients who progress on single-agent BRAF inhibitors appear to reactivate the RAF/MEK/ERK pathway in a number of proposed ways: acquired NRAS mutations; amplification of BRAF itself; expression of splice variants of BRAF that form active BRAF dimers; overexpression of MEK; or by mutations in MEK.[10,24,25] Methods to overcome these pathways of resistance will be discussed later in the chapter. It should be noted that single agent therapy with these agents are no longer the standard of care and combination treatment upfront to prevent resistance is now the standard. The combination strategy will be discussed later in this chapter.

Trametinib

Trametinib (Mekinist®) is an orally available small-molecule inhibitor of MEK1 and MEK2 that was approved by the FDA in May of 2013 for the treatment of BRAF-mutated melanoma. A multicenter randomized control trial in patients with stage IIIC and stage IV unresectable, histologically confirmed melanoma with confirmation of V600E or V600K mutation compared trametinib to dacarbazine. The study included some 322 patients, of whom 214 were assigned in a 2:1 ratio to receive oral trametinib (2 mg once daily) versus intravenous chemotherapy with either dacarbazine (1000 mg/m2) or paclitaxel (175 mg/m2) at the discretion of the investigator, given every three weeks. Results showed response rates of more than 20% in *BRAF*-mutated melanoma with a median progression-free survival of 4.8 months compared to 1.5 months for dacarbazine.[26]

Trametinib was well tolerated in the single-agent studies. The most common adverse events were diarrhea, skin rash, and ocular toxicity, including reversible central serous retinopathy. Ocular events (grade 1 and 2) occurred in roughly 9% of patients, with blurred vision the most frequently observed adverse event (4%). All patients should have a dilated eye examination before starting, and repeat examinations if they experience any visual changes. Decreased ejection fraction or ventricular dysfunction was observed in 7% of patients and was reversible with stopping the agent. Patients should have an ejection fraction evaluation prior to starting treatment, as well as if any symptoms of cardiac failure occur during treatment. The skin rash is typically an acne-form dermatitis that responds well to topical antibiotics and steroids. Dose reductions and drug holidays are effective in management of the more serious toxicities.

The real clinical question is when clinicians should use trametinib as a single agent in *BRAF*-mutated melanoma. Responses to this drug have not been seen in disease that has progressed on a *BRAF* inhibitor, and it should not be used in *BRAF* inhibitor–refractory cases. Though the two were not compared directly, the response rates to single-agent *BRAF* inhibitors appear to be higher than with MEK inhibition. Because of this, most believe that *BRAF* inhibitors such as vemurafenib and dabrafenib should be used over trametinib in unresectable,metastatic *BRAF*-mutated melanoma population.

Imatinib

The oncogene *KIT* is also a key player in the melanoma genome-activation pathway, particularly in mucosal and acral melanomas. Imatinib was studied in 295 patients with metastatic melanoma and demonstrated a response rate of 16%.[27,28] Other studies have seen higher response rates, particularly if the tumor has mutations in exon 11 or 12 of *KIT*. Overall, however, the efficacy of imatinib in *KIT*-mutated melanoma has been underwhelming, with the response rates being relatively low and of minimal durability.

Combination Therapy: Dabrafenib plus Trametinib

As previously discussed, early single-agent *BRAF* inhibitors are effective, but almost universal resistance develops in months. Given that reactivation of the MAPK pathway is paramount in resistance mechanisms, combination therapy with BRAF and MEK inhibitors is a very promising method to overcome resistance.[29] Dabrafenib and trametinib (CombiDT) was the first such combination to be clinically studied. In a randomized phase II study, 54 *BRAF*-mutant melanoma patients who received full-dose treatment with dabrafenib at 150 mg PO BID and trametinib at 2 mg PO QD had improved PFS and RR over patients treated with dabrafenib alone. The RR to the combination versus dabrafenib alone was 76% versus 54%, respectively, with a median PFS of 9.4 versus 5.8 months. The most impressive of these results was a median survival for Stage IV unresectable melanoma patients treated with dabrafenib and trametinib was 23.8 months.[30,31] Based on these data, the FDA approved dabrafenib and trametinib in combination for the treatment on of *BRAF* V600-mutated melanoma in January of 2014, contingent upon the successful completion of the phase III study. A recent press release by GlaxoSmithKline (GSK) announced that the phase III study showed statistically improved PFS of the combination over single-agent dabrafenib, and that the median overall survival results were similar to that seen in the phase II study.

Interestingly, the combination therapy tends to be less toxic than either agent alone. This decrease in toxicity has been attributed to MEK inhibitors' reducing the downstream consequences of paradoxical activation in *BRAF* wild-type keratinocytes; thus the combination would be predicted to, and does, result in a profound decrease in skin toxicities.[23] However it should be noted that pyrexia occurs in the majority of patients (76%) on the combination.[30] This can be managed by dose reductions as well as low-dose steroids (prednisone 10 mg daily) once infectious causes of fever have been eliminated.

Because of the improved toxicity profile and the improved overall outcomes, most experts believe that combination treatment should replace single-agent *BRAF* inhibitors.

Conclusion

Understanding of melanoma biology has directly led to drug development in melanoma and has drastically changed the landscape of this disease. More driver mutations are being identified, and drugs to block these new targets are under development. Further understanding of resistance mechanisms will lead to more combination trials, both with other signal transduction inhibitors as well as with immune therapies.

References

1. Tsai J, Lee JT, Wang W, et al. Discovery of a selective inhibitor of oncogenic B-Raf kinase with potent antimelanoma activity. *Proc Natl Acad Sci.* 2008;105(8):3041–3046.

2. Agrawal SS. Current systemic therapy for metastatic melanoma. *Expert Rev Anticancer Ther.* 2009;9:587–595.

3. Mar VJ, Wong SQ, Li J, et al. *BRAF/NRAS* wild-type melanomas have a high mutation load correlating with histologic and molecular signatures of UV damage. *Clin Cancer Res.* 19(17):4589–4598.

4. Schlessinger, J. Cell signaling by receptor tyrosine kinases. *Cell.* 2000;103(2):211–225.

5. Chang L, Karin M. Mammalian MAP kinase signalling cascades. *Nature.* 2001;410(6824):37–40.

6. Hanahan D, Weinberg RA. Hallmarks of cancer: the next generation. *Cell.* 2011;144(5):646–674.

7. Curtin JA, Busam K, Pikel D, Bastian BC. Somatic activation of *KIT* in distinct subtypes of melanoma. *J Clin Oncol.* 2006;24(26):4340–4346.

8. Flaherty KT, Hodi FS, Fisher DE. From genes to drugs: targeted strategies for melanoma. *Nat Rev Cancer.* 2012;12(5):349–361.

9. Furney SJ, Turaijlic S, Stamp G, et al. Genome sequencing of mucosal melanomas reveals that they are driven by distinct mechanisms from cutaneous melanoma. *J Pathol.* 2013;230(3):261–269.

10. Nazarian R, Shi H, Wang Q, et al. Melanomas acquire resistance to B-RAF(V600E) inhibition by RTK or N-RAS upregulation. *Nature.* 2010;468(7326):973–977.

11. Pollock PM, Harper UL, Hansen KS, et al. High frequency of *BRAF* mutations in nevi. *Nat Genet.* 2003;33:19–20.

12. Vultur A, Villanueva J, Herlyn M. Targeting *BRAF* in advanced melanoma: a first step toward manageable disease. *Clin Cancer Res.* 2011;17(7):1658–1663.

13. Davies H, Bignell GR, Cox C, et al. Mutations of the *BRAF* gene in human cancer. *Nature.* 2002; 417(6892):949–954.

14. Sharma A, Trivedi NR, Zimmeraman MA, et al. Mutant V599EB-Raf regulates growth and vascular development of malignant melanoma tumors. *Cancer Res.* 2005;65(6):2412–2421.

15. Landi MT, Bauer J, Pfeiffer RM, et al. MC1R germline variants confer risk for *BRAF*-mutant melanoma. *Science.* 2006;313(5786):521–522.

16. Salama AK, Flaherty KT. *BRAF* in melanoma: current strategies and future directions. *Clin Cancer Res.* 2013;19(16):4326–4334.

17. Bucheit AD, Syklawer E, Jakob JA, et al. Clinical characteristics and outcomes with specific *BRAF* and *NRAS* mutations in patients with metastatic melanoma. *Cancer.* 2013;119(21):3821–3829.

18. Flaherty KT, Puzanov I, Kim KB, et al. Inhibition of mutated, activated *BRAF* in metastatic melanoma. *N Engl J Med.* 2010;363(9):809–819.

19. Chapman PB, Hauschild A, Robert C, et al. Improved survival with vemurafenib in melanoma with *BRAF* V600E mutation. *N Engl J Med.* 2011;364(26): 2507–2516.

20. Sosman JA, Kim KB, Schuchter L, et al. Survival in *BRAF* V600-mutant advanced melanoma treated with vemurafenib. *N Engl J Med.* 2012;366(8):707–714.

21. Hauschild A, Grobb JJ, Demidov LV, et al. Dabrafenib in *BRAF*-mutated melanoma: a multicentre, open-label, phase 3 randomised controlled trial. *Lancet.* 2012;380(9839):358–365.

22. Acerkman A, Klein O, McDermott DF, et al. Outcomes of patients with metastatic melanoma treated with immunotherapy prior to or after *BRAF* inhibitors. *Cancer.* 2014; epub ahead of print. doi: 10.1002/cncr.28620.

23. Su F, Viros A, Milagre C, et al. *RAS* mutations in cutaneous squamous-cell carcinomas in patients treated with *BRAF* inhibitors. *N Engl J Med.* 2012;366(3):207–215.

24. McArthur G, Ribas A, Chapman P, et al. Molecular analyses from a phase I trial of vemurafenib to study mechanism of action (MOA) and resistance in repeated biopsies from *BRAF* mutation-positive metastatic melanoma patients (pts). *J Clin Oncol.* 2011;29(566s): abstr 8502.

25. Sosman J, Pavlick A, Schuchter L, et al: Analysis of molecular mechanisms of response and resistance to vemurafenib (vem) in BRAFV600E melanoma. *J Clin Oncol.* 2012;30(540s): abstr 8503.

26. Flaherty KT, Robert C, Hersey P, et al. Improved survival with *MEK* inhibition in *BRAF*-mutated melanoma. *N Engl J Med*. 2012;377:107–114.

27. Carvajal RD, Antonescu CR, Wolchok JD et al. *KIT* as a therapeutic target in metastatic melanoma. *JAMA*. 2011;305(22):2327–2334.

28. Guo J, Si L, Kong Y, et al. Phase II, open-label, single-arm trial of imatinib mesylate in patients with metastatic melanoma harboring *c-Kit* mutation or amplification. *J Clin Oncol*. 2011; 29(21):2904–2909.

29. Paraiso KH, Fedorenko IV, Cantini LP, et al. Recovery of phospho-ERK activity allows melanoma cells to escape from *BRAF* inhibitor therapy. *Br J Cancer*. 2010; 102(12):1724–1730.

30. Flaherty KT, Infante JR, Daud A, et al. Combined *BRAF* and *MEK* inhibition in melanoma with *BRAF V600* mutations. *N Engl J Med*. 2012;367(18):1694–1703.

31. Daud, Weber J, Sosam J, et al. Overall survival update of BRF113220 Part C, a Phase II three-arm randomized study of dabrafenib alone (D) vs. a combination of dabrafenib and trametinib (D + T) in patients with *BRAF V600* mutation-positive metastatic melanoma. Society for Melanoma Research, 2013: Philadelphia, PA, USA.

Chapter 10

The Role of Cytotoxic Chemotherapy in Melanoma

Adil Daud and Michelle Ashworth

Advanced (unresectable stage III, metastatic stage IV) melanoma is often described as being resistant to cytotoxic chemotherapy, with low objective response rates (complete response plus partial response) across regimens in various melanoma subtypes (cutaneous, mucosal, or uveal). As a result, chemotherapy has been largely palliative. Occasionally, however, a complete response occurs, or a deep partial response can be followed by metastectomy and lead to prolonged disease-free survival. This chapter will focus largely on the response rate and overall survival benefit offered by selected regimens, provide a brief historic overview of regimens evaluated in advanced melanoma, and discuss the regimens commonly in use today.

Historical Clinical Trials

It should be kept in mind that many historical clinical trials did not specify the melanoma subtype when reporting responses to treatment, and many trials specifically excluded patients with uveal melanoma; therefore, it is important to review available data with an eye to subtype whenever possible, and to give this information proper weight in treatment selection and in the design and publication of future clinical trials. In general, the vast majority of patients treated in clinical trials and discussed herein had advanced cutaneous melanoma, unless otherwise specified. When critically reviewing results of trials in patients with advanced melanoma, it is also key to note that patient inclusion and exclusion criteria can influence the observed response rate and overall survival attributed to a given regimen, with higher response rates often observed among treatment-naïve populations as compared to pretreated patients, and longer overall survival when patients with poor prognostic factors such as presence of brain metastases or elevated LDH are excluded.[1] Another common theme identifiable on review of these trials is a trend towards higher response rates among patients with metastases to lung and soft tissue, as compared to liver or bone.

Dacarbazine and Temozolomide

Dacarbazine (DTIC), approved by the U.S. Food and Drug Administration (FDA) in 1975 for the treatment of metastatic melanoma, is an intravenously administered DNA-alkylating agent metabolized via *N*-demethylation in the cytochrome p450 (CYP1A1, CYP1A2, and CYP2E1) system in the liver to its active species, 5-(3-methyl)1-trizen-1-yl-imidazole-4-carboxamide (MTIC).[2] Its activity is subject to interference by inhibitors of the p450 system. Dacarbazine does not penetrate the central nervous system (CNS).

Temozolomide (Temodar) is an orally bioavailable form of dacarbazine that does not require hepatic metabolism but rather breaks down in plasma via hydrolysis at physiological pH, is active within the central nervous system (CNS), and has been shown to have activity equivalent to that of dacarbazine in metastatic melanoma, with a similar toxicity profile.[3,4] Major methylated species formed by dacarbazine or temozolomide are N^7-methylguanine (70%), N^3-methyladenine (9.2%), and O^6-methylguanine (5%).[5] N^7-methylguanine and N^3-methyladenine are quickly remedied by base excision repair, leaving the minority of DNA damage, O^6-methylguanine, as the cytotoxic lesion. O^6-methylguanine lesions present at replication cause repetitive futile rounds of mismatch repair, and trigger apoptosis. However, O^6-methylguanine can be directly repaired by O^6-methylguanine-DNA methyltransferase (MGMT), and tumors with high levels of MGMT have been found to be resistant to alkylating agents.[6] Commonly used monotherapy regimens include dacarbazine 150–250 mg/m^2 intravenous daily on days 1–5 or 1000–1200 mg/m^2 IV d1 of a 21- or 28-day cycle, or temozolomide 200 mg/m^2 by mouth daily on days 1–5 of a 21-day cycle. Adverse effect profiles of both drugs include nausea requiring prophylactic antiemetic medication, and myelosuppression (at higher rates in geriatric patients) requiring monitoring of counts and in some cases dose modification. Dosing adjustment recommendations exist for the use of dacarbazine in patients with renal impairment, but not in those with hepatic dysfunction.[7] As its metabolism is peripheral, temozolomide may be used in patients with moderate renal or hepatic impairment, but it has not been studied in advanced renal or hepatic impairment.[8] In a recent meta-analysis of 48 trials featuring treatment with dacarbazine as a control arm (3,356 patients), overall response rate to dacarbazine monotherapy averaged 15.3% (range 5.3–28%), with lower response rates among larger or newer trials.[9] In the largest trial in the series ($n = 415$), overall survival among the few patients who responded to treatment was 12.4 months, vs. 3.75 mo for non-responders.[10] In the head-to-head comparison of dacarbazine to temozolomide in 280 patients, the response rate was 12.5% vs. 13.5%, and median overall survival was 6.4 mo vs. 7.7 mo (this difference did not reach statistical significance).[3]

Many dacarbazine-based multi-agent chemotherapy regimens have been evaluated, without significant improvement in overall survival compared to monotherapy, and with increased toxicity.[11,12] The medical literature is littered with acronym-bearing regimens that showed promise in phase II trials, but unfortunately these have not shown definitive superiority to dacarbazine in randomized phase III trials. One challenge in designing and administering combination cytotoxic chemotherapy regimens has been overlapping toxicity profiles; for example, chemotherapy agents are myelosuppressive to some extent, so combination chemotherapy regimens can lead to an increased response rate that does not correlate with improved median overall survival, due to excess toxicity. Also, with low response rates, a small number of patients may have sustained responses that are not sufficiently frequent to significantly influence median overall survival in the entire trial population.

BOLD Regimen

Treatment of 91 patients with the BOLD regimen (bleomycin 7.5–15 units subcut d1, 4; vincristine [aka Oncovin] 1 mg/m^2 IV d1, 5; lomustine 80 mg/m^2 PO d1; dacarbazine 200 mg/m^2 IV d1–5 of a 28-day cycle) resulted in a 32% response rate and overall survival of 7.2 months.[13] The addition of interferon-α-2b (IFN) (3 MU subcut d8–42, then 6 MU subcut 3x/week) to the BOLD regimen in 43 patients led to a response rate of 27% and median overall survival of 5 months.[14] To highlight the point previously made regarding the importance of accounting for patient characteristics when evaluating study outcomes, it is interesting to compare this trial, which included patients with stage IV disease (100%), brain metastases (22%), and prior chemotherapy (17%), to another trial of the BOLD plus IFN regimen in 48 patients, 46% of whom had stage III disease, 10% had brain metastases, and 8% had prior chemotherapy. This trial reported an overall response rate of 62%, which has not been duplicated.[15]

Dartmouth Regimen (CBDT)

The Dartmouth or CBDT regimen—with some variation in dosing across trials, generally cisplatin 25 mg/m^2 IV daily d1–3, carmustine (a.k.a. BCNU) 100–150 mg/m^2 IV d1 every other cycle, dacarbazine 220 mg/m^2 IV daily d1–3, and tamoxifen 10 mg PO BID or 40 mg PO QD on 21-day cycles—led to a response rate of 27% and median survival of 5.5 months in a phase II trial of 30 patients.[16] In a randomized phase II trial in 60 patients of CBDT vs. dacarbazine 1200 mg/m^2 IV d1 on a 21-day cycle, the response rates were 26% vs. 5%, respectively, with median overall survival of 9 mo vs. 7 mo; this was accompanied by 33% vs. 15% grade 3–4 myelotoxicity.[17] Another phase II trial comparing CBDT to CBD (tamoxifen vs. placebo) in 199 patients showed that the addition of tamoxifen to the regimen did not lead to a significant improvement in response rate (30% vs. 21%, $p = 0.187$) or overall survival (women, 7.75 mo vs. 8 mo, $p = 0.99$, men 7.25 mo vs. 7.25 mo, $p = 0.37$).[18] Finally, the large phase III trial of CBDT vs. dacarbazine 1000 mg/m^2 IV d1 on a 21-day cycle in 240 patients did not show a statistically significant difference in objective response rate (18.5% vs. 10.2%, $p = 0.09$) or median overall survival (7.7 mo vs. 6.4 mo, $p = 0.51$), and was accompanied by a 39% vs. 19% risk of grade 3–4 neutropenia, with one treatment-related death (cerebral hemorrhage due to thrombocytopenia).[19]

The Nitrosoureas

The nitrosoureas (e.g., fotemustine, lomustine, and carmustine), a class of alkylating agents that also have activity in the CNS, have demonstrated activity in advanced melanoma; in one study of 169 patients treated with *fotemustine* 100 mg/m^2 IV weekly x 3 weeks (induction) followed by a rest for 4–5 weeks, then 100 mg/m^2 IV every 3 weeks (maintenance), a response rate of 24.2% was seen.[20] However, in the phase III trial comparing this fotemustine regimen with dacarbazine 250 mg/m² IV daily d1–5/28 in 229 patients, the overall response rate was higher with fotemustine (15.2% vs. 6.8%, $p = 0.043$), but the median survival was not significantly improved (7.3 mo vs. 6.8 mo, $p = 0.067$).[20,21] As the nitrosoureas are notable for delayed-onset myelotoxicity and dose-related pulmonary toxicity, their use in advanced melanoma has not gained favor over other agents, and fotemustine is not available in the United States. In Europe, however, fotemustine has gained favor and is often used clinically in preference to or after dacarbazine.

Platinum-Based Drugs

Cisplatin and *carboplatin*, platinum-based intravenously administered chemotherapy drugs that covalently bind to DNA bases causing DNA cross-linking, denaturation, strand breakage and subsequent cell apoptosis, have each demonstrated activity as monotherapy in advanced melanoma, and are active in the CNS.

Cisplatin 100 mg/m² IV every 21 days led to an objective response rate of 10.4% (7/67) in one trial,[22] and in another 42 patients treated with cisplatin 120 mg/m² IV every 21 days, there was a 17% response rate and median overall survival of 7.6 months.[23] Cisplatin is notable for adverse effects, including nausea and vomiting, requiring prophylactic antiemetics such as steroids; neurotoxicity, ototoxicity, and nephrotoxicity requiring pretreatment IV hydration; it is contraindicated in renal impairment, but there are no dose-adjustment recommendations in the setting of hepatic dysfunction.[24]

Carboplatin has a markedly longer half-life and a different toxicity profile than cisplatin, with a higher risk of myelosuppression, slightly less emetogenesis, and much less neurotoxicity, ototoxicity, or nephrotoxicity; it does not require administration of pretreatment IV hydration. The currently used equation for calculating carboplatin dosing (Calvert formula for area under the curve, or AUC) incorporates an individual patient's renal function, and no dose-adjustment recommendations are provided for hepatic dysfunction.[25] A phase II study of carboplatin 400 mg/m² IV every 28 days in 43 patients showed a response rate of 16%,[26] and in another study of 30 patients led to a response rate of 11% with median overall survival of 4.7 months.[27] The reported efficacy of cisplatin or carboplatin monotherapy is modest, and comparable to historical data in dacarbazine and temozolomide. The selection of cisplatin vs. carboplatin can be aided by consideration of each drug's toxicity profile: for example, cisplatin is not a good choice in a patient with preexisting neuropathy, and carboplatin may not be well tolerated by a patient who has previously received chemotherapy or radiation treatment that resulted in depleted marrow reserves. As regards combination therapy, a trial in 28 patients of combination therapy with cisplatin 40 mg/m² IV daily d1–5 and dacarbazine 500 mg/m² IV daily d1–2 of a 28-day cycle was poorly tolerated, with grade 3–4 toxicity in 51% of treatment courses, and a response rate of 29%.[28] In another series of 62 patients treated with cisplatin 100 mg/m² and dacarbazine 750 mg/m² IV, there was a 14% response rate with 67% experiencing grade 3–4 toxicity.[29] Overall, this combination appears excessively toxic without establishing superiority to monotherapy.

Oxaliplatin has not been extensively evaluated in advanced melanoma; one patient was observed to have a response in a phase I trial,[30] and zero objective responses were observed when oxaliplatin was given in combination with docetaxel and GM-CSF in 14 evaluable patients.[31]

The Taxanes

The taxanes (e.g., docetaxel, paclitaxel, and *nab*-paclitaxel) are intravenously delivered antimitotic microtubule stabilizing agents with activity in advanced melanoma, but these are not effective within the CNS due to efflux back across the blood–brain barrier mediated by P-glycoprotein.[32–34] The toxicity profile of taxanes includes hypersensitivity reactions (with treatment protocols requiring premedication with antihistamines and corticosteroid in many trials), alopecia, myelosuppression, skin toxicities, and peripheral edema, as well as peripheral neuropathy and mucositis.

In a trial of *docetaxel* (Taxotere) 100 mg/m^2 IV every 21 days in 40 patients, a response rate of 12.5% was observed, with median overall survival of 13 mo[35]; in another trial, of 30 patients, objective response rate was 17%, and median survival was 6.5 months.[36] In both trials, enrollment was limited to chemotherapy-naïve patients without brain metastases. In 62 chemotherapy-naïve patients (including 8 with brain metastases) treated with docetaxel 80 mg/m^2 IV d1 plus temozolomide 150 mg/m^2 PO daily d1–5 on 28 day cycles, a response rate of 27% was observed, with median overall survival of 16 mo, with 25% grade 3–4 leukopenia.[37] Among 38 previously treated patients (42% with brain metastases) treated with this same regimen, the response rate was 13% and overall survival was 6.5 months.[38]

In a trial of 25 patients treated with *paclitaxel* (Taxol) 80 mg/m^2 IV weekly 3 out of 4 weeks, zero objective responses were observed.[39] However, in a trial of paclitaxel 90 mg/m^2 IV d1, 5, and 9 of a 21-day cycle in 32 patients, a response rate of 15.6% was observed,[40] and in 34 patients treated with paclitaxel 250 mg/m^2 IV every 21 days, the response rate was 14%, with two patients experiencing durable complete responses over 14 months.[41] This was complicated by 12% rate of anaphylactic reactions despite premedication.

Nab-paclitaxel (Abraxane) is an albumin-bound form of paclitaxel that is not delivered in the Cremophor base, which can be responsible for hypersensitivity reactions to paclitaxel. In a phase II trial of 74 patients treated with *nab*-paclitaxel 150 mg/m^2 (37 chemotherapy-naïve patients) or 100 mg/m^2 (37 pretreated patients) IV weekly 3 out of 4 weeks, a response rate of 21.6% in chemotherapy-naïve patients and 2.7% in pretreated patients was observed, with overall survival of 12.1 mo and 9.6 mo, respectively. Grade 3–4 neutropenia was seen in 41% vs. 14% of patients. In a phase III trial in 529 patients without brain metastases, directly comparing *nab*-paclitaxel 150 mg/m^2 IV d1, 8, and 15 of a 28-day cycle vs. dacarbazine 1000 mg/m^2 IV every 21 days, response rate was 15% vs. 11%, and overall survival was 12.8 mo vs. 10.7 mo ($p = 0.094$).[42] In another comparison of chemotherapy-naïve vs. pretreated patients treated with carboplatin AUC 2 plus *nab*-paclitaxel 100 mg/m^2 IV d1, 8, and 16 of 28-day cycles, response rate was 25.6% vs. 8.8%, with overall survival of 11.1 mo vs. 10.9 mo and grade 3–4 neutropenia in 28% and 41%.[43]

Current Mainstays of Treatment by Melanoma Type

After several decades of vigorous research into combination chemotherapy regimens, the mainstays of treatment with cytotoxic chemotherapy in advanced melanoma remain single-agent chemotherapy with dacarbazine, temozolomide, platinum, or taxane, or the fairly well-tolerated combination of carboplatin plus paclitaxel. As with other small trials in combination chemotherapy in melanoma, the data to back carboplatin plus paclitaxel have been mixed. In a trial of paclitaxel 100 mg/m^2 IV weekly vs. paclitaxel 80 mg/m^2 IV plus carboplatin 200 mg/m^2 IV weekly in previously treated patients, objective response rate was 2/18 (11%) vs. 0/16 with median overall survival of 7.5 mo vs. 7.8 months.[44] In a trial of carboplatin AUC 6 + paclitaxel 225 mg/m^2 every 21 days in 135 previously treated patients, the response rate was 12%, and median overall survival was 10.5 mo, with a 47% grade 3–4 toxicity rate.[45] In a large phase III trial in 823 chemotherapy-naïve patients comparing carboplatin AUC 6 + paclitaxel 225 mg/m^2 IV every 21 days with or without sorafenib 400 mg PO BID, response rate was 20% vs. 18%, and median overall survival rate was 11.3 mo vs. 11.1 mo, which indicated no additional benefit from sorafenib, but did supply efficacy data in a large number of patients for carboplatin plus paclitaxel.[46] Carboplatin AUC 6 + paclitaxel 225 mg/m^2 IV every 21 days is an oft-selected regimen in clinical practice and is currently in use as a standard of care comparator arm in the evaluation of new agents in clinical trials.

Metastatic Uveal Melanoma

Metastatic uveal melanoma, like cutaneous melanoma, is generally resistant to cytotoxic chemotherapy. In a review of 64 patients with metastatic uveal melanoma treated on a variety of chemotherapy-based Southwest Oncology Group (SWOG) trials during the 1980s, an overall response rate of 9% (6/64) was observed, vs. 11% in the trial patients with non-uveal melanoma.[47] Comparing patients with uveal melanoma metastatic to liver vs. metastatic to other sites, the response rate was 5% (3/57) vs. 43% (3/7)—a key piece of data, given that 89% of patients with uveal melanoma will present with metastases to the liver.[48]

In a group of 16 patients with uveal melanoma metastatic to the liver treated with CBDT, a 6% (1/21) objective response rate was seen.[49] The following results were all found in patients with metastatic uveal melanoma. Among 4 patients on a pilot study of liposomal vincristine sulfate 2 mg/m^2 every 14 days, one response was seen.[50] In a phase II trial of treatment with DHA-paclitaxel 150 mg/m^2 IV weekly, response was seen in 4.5% (1/22) patients,[51] and in a phase II trial of treatment with temozolomide 75 mg/m^2 d1–21/28 in 14 patients with metastatic uveal melanoma, zero objective responses were observed.[52]

The BOLD plus IFN regimen described above was administered in a multicenter trial to 21 patients with metastatic uveal melanoma, and zero objective responses were observed.[53] In a trial of 24 patients with uveal melanoma treated with sorafenib 400 mg PO BID, carboplatin AUC 6, and paclitaxel 225 mg/m^2 IV on 21-day cycles, zero objective responses were observed, and median OS was 11 months.[54]

As with cutaneous melanoma, agents that showed promise in early trials have not proven effective in repeated studies,[55–58] and trials are slow to accrue with small numbers in this rare disease. Despite the low response rates, since stable disease and rare objective responses can be observed, many patients with metastatic uveal melanoma are still offered palliative-intent treatment with cytotoxic chemotherapy. Given the dismal responses to chemotherapy to date, treatment with targeted therapy (e.g., MEK inhibitors) and liver-directed therapy are areas of active research, and metastatic uveal melanoma remains a disease with an active need for therapeutic innovation. The best option for a patient with metastatic uveal melanoma remains referral for evaluation for enrollment onto clinical trial, where appropriate and available.

Metastatic Mucosal Melanoma

As with uveal melanoma, because advanced mucosal melanoma is a rare subtype of melanoma, trials specifically for patients with advanced mucosal melanoma can be difficult to complete and slow to accrue, and patients with mucosal melanoma may be included in trials of patients with cutaneous melanoma, but their outcomes may not be reported separately. In the adjuvant setting (resected stage II–III mucosal melanoma), a recent trial in 189 patients of post-surgical observation vs. high-dose interferon (HD-IFN) vs. temozolomide 200 mg/m^2 PO d1–5 + cisplatin 75 mg/m^2 IV given in divided doses d1–3 of 21-day cycles for 6 cycles, resulted in median overall survival of 21.2, 40.4, and 48.7 mo, respectively, with relapse-free survival of 5.4, 9.4, and 20.8 mo,[59] indicating a benefit in the adjuvant setting that may well translate into benefit in the metastatic setting, but as there are not clear data to support this to date, targeted therapy and immunotherapy are important areas of active research.

Biochemotherapy

Multi-agent chemotherapy in combination with cytokine therapy, also known as biochemotherapy (BCT), has resulted in higher reported response rates. In a trial comparing dacarbazine plus interferon (IFN) vs. the BOLD regimen plus IFN (evaluating natural IFN-α vs. recombinant interferon α-2b), response rate was 8–12% in the dacarbazine plus IFN arms and 13–24% in the BOLD plus IFN arms (differences did not reach statistical significance), and overall survival was 9.1–11.1 mo in the dacarbazine plus IFN arms and 7.5–9.8 mo in the BOLD plus IFN arms, with increased toxicity in the BOLD-containing arms.[60]

More recently, Legha and coworkers at MD Anderson Cancer Center pioneered CVD-based biochemotherapy regimens.[61] In their initial trial, 40 *highly selected* patients treated with CVD (cisplatin 20 mg/m^2 IV daily d1–4, vinblastine 1.2 mg/m^2 IV daily d1–4, and dacarbazine 800 mg/m^2 IV d1) + interleukin-2 (IL-2) 9 MIU/m^2 IV per day as continuous IV infusion d1–4)

+ interferon-alpha (IFN-α) 5 MU/m^2 subcut daily d1–5, 8, 10, and 12 for a maximum of four cycles, with maximal protocol-driven support with growth factors, prophylactic antibiotics, and vasopressors as needed, a response rate of 48% and median survival of 11 months was observed, with a significant toxicity profile including neutropenic fever in 64%, bacteremia in 49%, and hypotension in 39%.[62] Based on this initial phase II trial, five randomized trials comparing BCT to chemotherapy alone have been conducted. The largest was ECOG E3695, which was associated with a higher response rate with BCT (19.5% vs. 13.8%, $p = 0.14$), but no advantage in overall survival (9 mo vs. 8.7 mo) or one-year survival (41% vs. 36.9%).[63] Biochemotherapy carries an increased burden of toxicity without an established benefit in overall survival compared to chemotherapy.[64,65] However, cytokine therapy is still useful in highly selected patient populations and can lead to long-term responses in a minority of patients, as discussed in another chapter.[66]

Predictive Biomarkers for Cytotoxic Chemotherapy in Advanced Melanoma

There are no predictive biomarkers in routine clinical use in the selection of cytotoxic chemotherapy treatments for patients with advanced melanoma, and this remains an area of active clinical research. Hypermethylation of the MGMT-promoter correlates with response to temozolomide in patients with glioblastoma,[67] and is being examined in advanced cutaneous melanoma,[68] but its effectiveness has not been borne out in treatment of metastatic uveal melanoma with alkylating agents.[69]

Regenerating gene 1A (REG1A) plays a role in tissue regeneration and cell proliferation in tumors of epithelial origin. In one study, lymph node metastasis tissue microarrays from 27 patients with stage III cutaneous melanoma treated with adjuvant chemotherapy were examined for correlation between REG1A protein expression and prognosis.[70] High REG1A expression correlated with improved prognosis among patients treated with chemotherapy ($p = 0.0013$), but correlated with worse outcomes in untreated patients. Melanoma cell lines with high REG1A expression showed greater sensitivity to dacarbazine (DTIC) and cisplatin, indicating a possible future role of REG1A expression as a predictive biomarker for chemosensitivity in cutaneous melanoma.

Chemopotentiation: Cytotoxic Chemotherapy and Other Agents

In an effort to increase efficacy while avoiding overlapping toxicities, combinations of cytotoxic chemotherapy with other agents designed to potentiate DNA damage or attack other targets in cell-proliferation pathways is an area of ongoing research. Poly-ADP ribose polymerase (PARP) is a DNA-damage-activated nuclear enzyme that plays a key signaling role in the base excision repair pathway.[71] The combination of a PARP inhibitor that will inhibit base excision repair with cytotoxic chemotherapy that causes DNA damage has been explored in advanced melanoma: in a study of 46 patients treated with PARP inhibitor rucaparib 12 mg/m^2 IV d1 + temozolomide 200 mg/m^2 PO daily, response rate was 17.4%, and median overall survival was 9.9 months.[72] Lomeguatrib, an inhibitor of O6-alkylguanine-DNA-alkyltransferase (AGT, a.k.a. MGMT), showed an ability to deplete MGMT, but this did not translate into clinical benefit when given in combination with temozolomide in a randomized phase II study in metastatic melanoma.[73,74] Sorafenib, a small-molecule kinase inhibitor *in vitro* of *VEGF*, *BRAF*, and *CRAF*, has not shown improvement in overall survival when given in combination with carboplatin plus paclitaxel in advanced melanoma; this regimen showed zero response in metastatic uveal melanoma.[45,54] Oblimersen, an anti-sense oligonucleotide to bcl-2 (an anti-apoptotic protein over-expressed in human cancers), was given as a continuous IV infusion 7 mg/kg/day or 900 mg/m^2 x 7 days d1–7 and 22–28 with temozolomide 75 mg/m^2 PO d1–42 and *nab*-paclitaxel 175 mg/m^2 or 260 mg/m^2 IV on d7 and d28 in a 56-day cycle in a phase I trial of 32 patients. This trial reported a response rate of 40.6% and median overall survival of 12 months, but patients with elevated LDH, brain metastases, or prior treatment were excluded.[75]

Conclusion

In summary, despite low response rates, for patients who have progressed after, or are not good candidates for, other appropriate agents (targeted therapy or immunotherapy), patients with advanced melanoma can be offered palliative-intent cytotoxic chemotherapy in hopes of achieving stable disease, relief from symptomatic disease, and improvement in quality of life; and with less frequency, an objective and possibly even a sustained response. Future advances in our understanding of the mechanisms of chemoresistance and discovery of appropriate combination regimens with improved efficacy and tolerability profiles will enhance the utility of chemotherapy in advanced melanoma.

In terms of choosing the specific chemotherapy regimen, at our center we use only a few of the regimens described above. In patients who have a good performance status and organ function, we use carboplatin/paclitaxel; and in all other patients, we use temozolomide. Other types of regimens that use nitrosoureas are not commonly used any more, as they tend to cause long-term bone marrow suppression. In cases where carboplatin/paclitaxel is not appropriate, the CVD regimen is most commonly employed as a reasonable combination regimen that does not contain a taxane. We recommend that most multispecialty practices use a few selected regimens, and that they thoroughly understand the toxicities and dose modifications of these regimens.

References

1. Korn EL, et al. Meta-analysis of phase II cooperative group trials in metastatic stage IV melanoma to determine progression-free and overall survival benchmarks for future phase II trials. *J Clin Oncol.* 2008;26(4):527–534.

2. Reid JM, et al. Metabolic activation of dacarbazine by human cytochromes P450: the role of CYP1A1, CYP1A2, and CYP2E1. *Clin Cancer Res.* 1999;5(8):2192–2197.

3. Middleton MR, et al. Randomized phase III study of temozolomide versus dacarbazine in the treatment of patients with advanced metastatic malignant melanoma. *J Clin Oncol.* 2000;18(1):158–166.

4. Patel PM, et al. Extended schedule, escalated dose temozolomide versus dacarbazine in stage IV melanoma: final results of a randomised phase III study (EORTC 18032). *Eur J Cancer.* 2011;47(10):1476–1483.

5. Newlands ES, et al. Temozolomide: a review of its discovery, chemical properties, pre-clinical development and clinical trials. *Cancer Treat Rev.* 1997;23(1):35–61.

6. Margison GP, Santibanez Koref MF, Povey AC. Mechanisms of carcinogenicity/chemotherapy by O6-methylguanine. *Mutagenesis.* 2002;17(6):483–487.

7. Dacarbazine: Drug Information. October 4, 2013. Available from: http://www.uptodate.com/contents/dacarbazine-drug-information.

8. Highlights of Prescribing Information: Temozolomide. October 4, 2013. Available from: http://www.merck.com/product/usa/pi_circulars/t/temodar_capsules/temodar_pi.pdf.

9. Lui P, et al. Treatments for metastatic melanoma: synthesis of evidence from randomized trials. *Cancer Treat Rev.* 2007;33(8):665–680.

10. Costanza ME, et al. Results with methyl-CCNU and DTIC in metastatic melanoma. *Cancer.* 1977;40(3):1010–1015.

11. Blesa JM, et al. Treatment options for metastatic melanoma: A systematic review. *Cancer Therapy.* 2009;7:188–199.

12. Serrone L, et al. Dacarbazine-based chemotherapy for metastatic melanoma: thirty-year experience overview. *J Exp Clin Cancer Res.* 2000;19(1):21–34.

13. Seigler HF, et al. DTIC, CCNU, bleomycin and vincristine (BOLD) in metastatic melanoma. *Cancer.* 1980;46(11):2346–2348.

14. Punt CJ, et al. Chemoimmunotherapy with bleomycin, vincristine, lomustine, dacarbazine (BOLD) plus interferon alpha for metastatic melanoma: a multicentre phase II study. *Br J Cancer.* 1997;76(2):266–269.

15. Pyrhonen S, Hahka-Kemppinen M, Muhonen T. A promising interferon plus four-drug chemotherapy regimen for metastatic melanoma. *J Clin Oncol.* 1992;10(12):1919–1926.

16. Johnston SR, et al. Randomized phase II trial of BCDT [carmustine (BCNU), cisplatin, dacarbazine (DTIC) and tamoxifen] with or without interferon alpha (IFN-alpha) and interleukin (IL-2) in patients with metastatic melanoma. *Br J Cancer.* 1998;77(8):1280–1286.

17. Chiarion Sileni V, et al. Phase II randomized study of dacarbazine, carmustine, cisplatin and tamoxifen versus dacarbazine alone in advanced melanoma patients. *Melanoma Res.* 2001;11(2):189–196.

18. Rusthoven JJ, et al. Randomized, double-blind, placebo-controlled trial comparing the response rates of carmustine, dacarbazine, and cisplatin with and without tamoxifen in patients with metastatic melanoma. National Cancer Institute of Canada Clinical Trials Group. *J Clin Oncol.* 1996;14(7):2083–2090.

19. Chapman PB, et al. Phase III multicenter randomized trial of the Dartmouth regimen versus dacarbazine in patients with metastatic melanoma. *J Clin Oncol.* 1999;17(9):2745–2751.

20. Jacquillat C, et al. Final report of the French multicenter phase II study of the nitrosourea fotemustine in 153 evaluable patients with disseminated malignant melanoma including patients with cerebral metastases. *Cancer*. 1990;66(9):1873–1878.

21. Avril MF, et al. Fotemustine compared with dacarbazine in patients with disseminated malignant melanoma: a phase III study. *J Clin Oncol*. 2004;22(6):1118–1125.

22. Al-Sarraf M, et al. Cisplatin hydration with and without mannitol diuresis in refractory disseminated malignant melanoma: a Southwest Oncology Group study. *Cancer Treat Rep*. 1982;66(1):31–35.

23. Glover D, et al. Phase II randomized trial of cisplatin and WR-2721 versus cisplatin alone for metastatic melanoma: an Eastern Cooperative Oncology Group study (E1686). *Melanoma Res*. 2003;13(6):619–626.

24. Cisplatin: Drug Information. October 6, 2013. Available from: http://www.uptodate.com/contents/cisplatin-drug-information.

25. Carboplatin: Drug Information. October 6, 2013. Available from: http://www.uptodate.com/contents/carboplatin-drug-information.

26. Casper ES, Bajorin D. Phase II trial of carboplatin in patients with advanced melanoma. *Invest New Drugs*. 1990;8(2):187–190.

27. Chang A, et al. Phase II trial of carboplatin in patients with metastatic malignant melanoma. A report from the Eastern Cooperative Oncology Group. *Am J Clin Oncol*. 1993;16(2):152–155.

28. Luger SM, et al. High-dose cisplatin and dacarbazine in the treatment of metastatic melanoma. *JNCI*. 1990;82(24):1934–1937.

29. Fletcher WS, et al. Evaluation of cisplatin and DTIC in inoperable stage III and IV melanoma. A Southwest Oncology Group study. *Am J Clin Oncol*. 1993;16(4):359–362.

30. Mathe G, et al. A phase I trial of trans-1-diaminocyclohexane oxalato-platinum (I-OHP). *Biomed Pharmacother*. 1986;40(10):372–376.

31. Locke F, Clark JI, Gajewski TF. A phase II study of oxaliplatin, docetaxel, and GM-CSF in patients with previously treated advanced melanoma. *Cancer Chemother Pharmacol*. 2010;65(3):509–514.

32. Rice A, et al. Overcoming the blood-brain barrier to taxane delivery for neurodegenerative diseases and brain tumors. *J Mol Neurosci*. 2003;20(3):339–343.

33. Fellner S, et al. Transport of paclitaxel (Taxol) across the blood-brain barrier in vitro and in vivo. *J Clin Invest*. 2002;110(9):1309–1318.

34. Vishnu P, Roy V. Safety and efficacy of *nab*-paclitaxel in the treatment of patients with breast cancer. 2011; Available from: http://www.la-press.com.

35. Bedikian AY, et al. Phase II trial of docetaxel in patients with advanced cutaneous malignant melanoma previously untreated with chemotherapy. *J Clin Oncol*. 1995;13(12):2895–2899.

36. Aamdal S, et al. Docetaxel (Taxotere) in advanced malignant melanoma: a phase II study of the EORTC Early Clinical Trials Group. *Eur J Cancer*. 1994;30A(8):1061–1064.

37. Bafaloukos D, et al. Temozolomide in combination with docetaxel in patients with advanced melanoma: a phase II study of the Hellenic Cooperative Oncology Group. *J Clin Oncol*. 2002;20(2):420–425.

38. Yoon C, et al. The clinical efficacy of combination of docetaxel and temozolomide in previously treated patients with stage IV melanoma. *Melanoma Res*. 2010;20(1):43–47.

39. Walker L, et al. Phase II trial of weekly paclitaxel in patients with advanced melanoma. *Melanoma Res.* 2005;15(5):453–459.

40. Bedikian AY, et al. Phase II evaluation of paclitaxel by short intravenous infusion in metastatic melanoma. *Melanoma Res.* 2004;14(1):63–66.

41. Einzig AI, et al. A phase II study of taxol in patients with malignant melanoma. *Invest New Drugs.* 1991;9(1):59–64.

42. Hersh E, Del Vecchio M, Brown M. Phase 3, randomized, open-label, multicenter trial of *nab*-paclitaxel versus dacarbazine in previously untreated patients with metastatic malignant melanoma. *Pigment Cell Melanoma Res.* 2012;25(6):863.

43. Kottschade LA, et al. A phase II trial of *nab*-paclitaxel (ABI-007) and carboplatin in patients with unresectable stage IV melanoma: a North Central Cancer Treatment Group Study, N057E(1). *Cancer.* 2011; 117(8):1704–1710.

44. Zimpfer-Rechner C, et al. Randomized phase II study of weekly paclitaxel versus paclitaxel and carboplatin as second-line therapy in disseminated melanoma: a multicentre trial of the Dermatologic Co-operative Oncology Group (DeCOG). *Melanoma Res.* 2003;13(5):531–536.

45. Hauschild A, et al. Results of a phase III, randomized, placebo-controlled study of sorafenib in combination with carboplatin and paclitaxel as second-line treatment in patients with unresectable stage III or stage IV melanoma. *J Clin Oncol.* 2009;27(17):2823–2830.

46. Flaherty KT, et al. Phase III trial of carboplatin and paclitaxel with or without sorafenib in metastatic melanoma. *J Clin Oncol.* 2013;31(3):373–379.

47. Flaherty LE, et al. Metastatic melanoma from intraocular primary tumors: the Southwest Oncology Group experience in phase II advanced melanoma clinical trials. *Am J Clin Oncol.* 1998;21(6):568–572.

48. Diener-West M, et al. Development of metastatic disease after enrollment in the COMS trials for treatment of choroidal melanoma: Collaborative Ocular Melanoma Study Group Report No. 26. *Arch Ophthalmol.* 2005;123(12):1639–1643.

49. F.E., N., et al. Response to combination chemotherapy of liver metastases from choroidal melanoma compared with cutaneous melanoma [Abstract]. *Proc Am Soc Clin Oncol.* 1994;13:396.

50. Bedikian AY, et al. A pilot study with vincristine sulfate liposome infusion in patients with metastatic melanoma. *Melanoma Res.* 2008;18(6):400–404.

51. Homsi J, et al. Phase 2 open-label study of weekly docosahexaenoic acid-paclitaxel in patients with metastatic uveal melanoma. *Melanoma Res.* 2010;20(6):507–510.

52. Bedikian AY, et al. Phase II evaluation of temozolomide in metastatic choroidal melanoma. *Melanoma Res.* 2003;13(3):303–306.

53. Kivela T, et al. Bleomycin, vincristine, lomustine and dacarbazine (BOLD) in combination with recombinant interferon alpha-2b for metastatic uveal melanoma. *Eur J Cancer.* 2003;39(8):1115–1120.

54. Bhatia S, et al. Phase II trial of sorafenib in combination with carboplatin and paclitaxel in patients with metastatic uveal melanoma: SWOG S0512. *PLoS One.* 2012;7(11):e48787.

55. Pfohler C, et al. Treosulfan and gemcitabine in metastatic uveal melanoma patients: results of a multicenter feasibility study. *Anticancer Drugs.* 2003;14(5):337–340.

56. Schmittel A, et al. Phase II trial of cisplatin, gemcitabine and treosulfan in patients with metastatic uveal melanoma. *Melanoma Res.* 2005;15(3):205–207.

57. Schmittel A, et al. A two-cohort phase II clinical trial of gemcitabine plus treosulfan in patients with metastatic uveal melanoma. *Melanoma Res.* 2005;15(5):447–451.

58. Schmittel A, et al. A randomized phase II trial of gemcitabine plus treosulfan versus treosulfan alone in patients with metastatic uveal melanoma. *Ann Oncol.* 2006;17(12):1826–1829.

59. Lian B, et al. Phase II randomized trial comparing high-dose IFN-alpha2b with temozolomide plus cisplatin as systemic adjuvant therapy for resected mucosal melanoma. *Clin Cancer Res.* 2013;19(16):4488–4498.

60. Vuoristo MS, et al. Randomized trial of dacarbazine versus bleomycin, vincristine, lomustine and dacarbazine (BOLD) chemotherapy combined with natural or recombinant interferon-alpha in patients with advanced melanoma. *Melanoma Res.* 2005;15(4):291–296.

61. Legha SS, et al. Development and results of biochemotherapy in metastatic melanoma: the University of Texas M.D. Anderson Cancer Center experience. *Cancer J Sci Am.* 1997;3(Suppl 1):S9–S15.

62. McDermott DF, et al. A phase II pilot trial of concurrent biochemotherapy with cisplatin, vinblastine, dacarbazine, interleukin 2, and interferon alpha-2B in patients with metastatic melanoma. *Clin Cancer Res.* 2000;6(6):2201–2208.

63. Atkins MB, et al. Phase III trial comparing concurrent biochemotherapy with cisplatin, vinblastine, dacarbazine, interleukin-2, and interferon alfa-2b with cisplatin, vinblastine, and dacarbazine alone in patients with metastatic malignant melanoma (E3695): a trial coordinated by the Eastern Cooperative Oncology Group. *J Clin Oncol.* 2008;26(35):5748–5754.

64. Sasse AD, et al. Chemoimmunotherapy versus chemotherapy for metastatic malignant melanoma. *Cochrane Database Syst Rev.* 2007(1):CD005413.

65. Ives NJ, et al. Chemotherapy compared with biochemotherapy for the treatment of metastatic melanoma: a meta-analysis of 18 trials involving 2,621 patients. *J Clin Oncol.* 2007;25(34):5426–5434.

66. Rosenberg SA, et al. Treatment of 283 consecutive patients with metastatic melanoma or renal cell cancer using high-dose bolus interleukin 2. *JAMA.* 1994;271(12):907–913.

67. Hegi ME, et al. Correlation of O6-methylguanine methyltransferase (MGMT) promoter methylation with clinical outcomes in glioblastoma and clinical strategies to modulate MGMT activity. *J Clin Oncol.* 2008;26(25):4189–4199.

68. Schraml P, et al. Predictive value of the MGMT promoter methylation status in metastatic melanoma patients receiving first-line temozolomide plus bevacizumab in the trial SAKK 50/07. *Oncol Rep.* 2012;28(2):654–658.

69. Voelter V, et al. Infrequent promoter methylation of the MGMT gene in liver metastases from uveal melanoma. *Int J Cancer.* 2008;123(5):1215–1218.

70. Sato Y, et al. Epigenetic regulation of *REG1A* and chemosensitivity of cutaneous melanoma. *Epigenetics.* 2013;8(10).

71. de Murcia G, Menissier de Murcia J. Poly(ADP-ribose) polymerase: a molecular nick-sensor. *Trends Biochem Sci.* 1994;19(4):172–176.

72. Plummer R, et al. A phase II study of the potent PARP inhibitor, Rucaparib (PF-01367338, AG014699), with temozolomide in patients with metastatic melanoma demonstrating evidence of chemopotentiation. *Cancer Chemother Pharmacol.* 2013;71(5):1191–1199.

73. Ranson M, et al. Lomeguatrib, a potent inhibitor of O6-alkylguanine-DNA-alkyltransferase; phase I safety, pharmacodynamic, and pharmacokinetic trial and evaluation in combination with temozolomide in patients with advanced solid tumors. *Clin Cancer Res.* 2006;12(5):1577–1584.

74. Ranson M, et al. Randomized trial of the combination of lomeguatrib and temozolomide compared with temozolomide alone in chemotherapy naïve patients with metastatic cutaneous melanoma. *J Clin Oncol.* 2007;25(18):2540–2545.

75. Ott PA, et al. Oblimersen in combination with temozolomide and albumin-bound paclitaxel in patients with advanced melanoma: a phase I trial. *Cancer Chemother Pharmacol.* 2013;71(1):183–191.

Chapter 11

Management of Melanoma Brain Metastases

Solmaz Sahebjam, Nikhil G. Rao, and Peter A. Forsyth

Melanoma commonly metastasizes to the brain and central nervous system (CNS); CNS metastases occur in more than 50% of patients with advanced melanoma.[1,2] This remarkable neurotropism has not yet been explained. The prognosis of patients with melanoma brain metastasis remains grim, and the median overall survival after diagnosis of brain metastases is only 2–9 months.[2–4] More brain metastases (>3), a lower Karnofsky performance score (KPS < 70), and higher levels of serum lactate dehydrogenase are associated with a poorer prognosis in this group of patients.[5,6]

We believe that the optimal management of melanoma brain metastasis patients requires the multidisciplinary collaboration of neurosurgeons, radiation oncologists, neuro-oncologists, and medical oncologists to tailor the treatment plan based on the clinical condition of the patient and the molecular characteristics of the tumor. Ideally, this should be based on a dedicated melanoma brain metastases clinic. We discuss each of the individual treatment modalities below.

Surgery

Surgical resection is one of the most effective treatment modalities for selected melanoma patients with brain metastases. Although there is no randomized trial evaluating the efficacy of surgery (nor is one likely to be performed), two large retrospective studies have reported significant improvement in the overall survival of patients with melanoma brain metastases who had surgical resection.[3,7] In one retrospective study, the median overall survival of patients who were treated with surgery was significantly longer than that of the non-surgical group (P value < 0.0001). Median survival for patients who were treated with surgery and radiotherapy or surgery alone was 8.9 and 8.7 months, respectively. The non-surgical group had a much shorter median survival (3.4 months for radiotherapy and 2.1 months for supportive care alone).[3] However, one must remember that a strong selection bias is inherent in these retrospective studies, and patients who underwent surgery were likely to have been selected for their limited intracranial and extracranial disease and good neurological functioning.

A randomized trial investigating use of surgery in patients with single brain metastasis from solid tumors (few had melanoma brain metastases) found a significant survival benefit in patients with controlled extracranial disease.[8] In this trial, 66 patients with a single brain metastasis from a solid tumor were entered in a randomized trial of neurosurgery plus whole-brain radiotherapy vs. whole-brain radiotherapy alone. Six out of 66 (9%) patients had melanoma brain metastasis. Combined treatment resulted in better survival (median 10 vs. 6 months; $P = 0.04$). Patients with inactive extracranial disease derived more benefit from combined treatment compared to radiation therapy alone (median 12 vs. 7 months; $P = 0.02$).[8]

In the aggregate, these data support the use of surgery in patients with limited intracranial disease and a favorable prognosis.[3,7,8]

Radiation Therapy

Whole-Brain Radiotherapy

Melanoma brain metastases are relatively radioresistant to whole-brain radiotherapy (WBRT).[9,10] Studies have combined WBRT with cytotoxic agents to improve its efficacy, such as fotemustine and temozolomide, but these have not improved its efficacy in comparison to WBRT as monotherapy.[9,11,12] For example, a randomized phase III trial of fotemustine plus WBRT (total dose of 37.5 Gray [Gy]) versus fotemustine alone in patients with melanoma brain metastases did not show any significant improvement in overall survival or local control rates.[11]

Moreover, available data do not support the use of WBRT after surgical resection of melanoma brain metastases. For example, in one retrospective study, there was no significant difference in the median survival between the 158 patients treated with surgery and WBRT versus the 47 patients treated with surgery alone (8.9 months vs. 8.7 months, $P = 0.21$).[3] Similar results in other retrospective studies have been found.[7]

For these reasons, we suggest that WBRT be reserved for patients who have large or symptomatic lesions, or those with multiple brain metastases that are not amenable to surgical resection, stereotactic radiosurgery, or systemic targeted (e.g., a BRAF inhibitor in a V600 mutant BRAF patient), or immunological therapy (e.g., a patient with multiple, very small, asymptomatic lesions and who does not require corticosteroids; see discussion below).

Stereotactic Radiosurgery

Stereotactic radiosurgery (SRS) is effective in achieving local control of melanoma brain metastases, with local control rates ranging from 81% to 97%.[6,10,13–15] Its effectiveness for local control and in improving survival are functions of both individual tumor volume and the total volume of SRS-treated brain metastases.[15,16] A small total tumor volume (<5 cc) and low number of intracranial metastases (i.e., <9 brain metastases) have been associated with improved local control and prolonged survival.[10,15] Therefore we do not recommend treating patients with SRS if the total tumor volume is ≥5 cm^3 or they have 10 or more brain metastases.

The substitution of post-resection SRS targeting the operative cavity instead of WBRT has been studied in several retrospective reviews of brain metastases from solid tumors in which local control rates were comparable to, or better than, WBRT.[17–19] Preoperative tumor diameters >3 cm and a lower conformality index have been associated with higher rates of local failure.[17,18] However, these studies are mainly from non-melanoma patients, and melanoma- specific studies are warranted given the unique biology of melanoma in the brain and the emergence of effective systemic therapy for melanoma.

Since melanoma has a higher risk of failure in distant brain sites after SRS than metastases from other solid tumors (Hazard Ratio [HR] 0.43; 95% confidence interval [CI] 0.19–0.95; P value = 0.038), it has been suggested that WRBT should follow SRS as a strategy to decrease the occurrence of brain metastases at sites that are "distant" from the SRS-treated site.[19] A randomized phase III trial recently investigated the role of WBRT after either surgery or SRS in patients with one to three brain metastases from solid tumors, though only 18 of the 359 (5%) randomized patients had melanoma brain metastases. Following local therapy with SRS or surgery, patients were randomly assigned to either WBRT or observation only. Although WBRT significantly reduced the two-year relapse rate both at initial sites (surgery: 59% to 27%, P value < 0.001; radiosurgery: 31% to 19%, P value − 0.040) and at new sites (surgery: 42% to 23%, P value = 0.008; radiosurgery: 48% to 33%, P value = 0.023), it did not improve the time to deterioration of performance status (primary endpoint of the study) or overall survival.[20] Similar results were found in another phase III trial that randomly assigned 132 patients with one to four brain metastases from solid tumors to SRS alone (18 to 25 Gy) or to SRS plus WBRT (30 Gy in 3-Gy fractions). WBRT resulted in an increase in both local and distant brain control, but with no improvement in overall survival.[21] However, the addition of WRBT to SRS was associated with a significant decline in cognitive function compared to SRS alone (mean posterior probability of decline, 52% vs. 24%, respectively). Therefore, the detrimental effect of WBRT on cognitive capacity and quality of life needs to be carefully considered before using WBRT after SRS.[22]

Systemic Therapy

Chemotherapy

Systemic treatment with cytotoxic chemotherapy has been largely ineffective in patients with melanoma brain metastases.[11,23,24] Trials of temozolomide and fotemustine, two compounds that penetrate the blood–brain barrier at therapeutically relevant concentrations, have shown no clinically meaningful efficacy. Their response rates are less than 10%.[11,23,24] Given the encouraging results of new targeted and immuno-therapies, the routine use of cytotoxic chemotherapy agents is not recommended for melanoma brain metastases.

Targeted Therapy for Melanoma Brain Metastasis

BRAF Inhibitors

Activating mutations of *BRAF* and *NRAS* have been associated with significantly higher risk of CNS metastases.[25] Several case reports have shown the efficacy of *BRAF* inhibitors in V600E *BRAF* mutant melanoma brain metastases and leptomeningeal involvement.[26–28] Hence, there has been a great deal of interest in evaluating the activity of *BRAF* inhibitors in melanoma brain metastases. To date, results of three clinical trials of small-molecule *BRAF* inhibitors in patients with melanoma brain metastases are available.[29,30] Furthermore, there is emerging evidence suggesting the efficacy of these agents in patients with tumors harboring V600 *BRAF* mutations other than V600E.[29,31,32]

Dabrafenib

A phase I/II study of dabrafenib included a cohort of 10 patients with asymptomatic untreated V600E and V600K *BRAF*-mutant melanoma.[30] A reduction in size of brain metastases was observed in 9 (90%) patients. Four (40%) patients achieved complete responses.[30] The encouraging results of this study led to the BREAK-MB phase II trial, which enrolled 172 patients with V600E or V600K *BRAF* mutant melanoma and active brain metastases.[29] Patients with one to four active melanoma brain metastases (≥5 mm to ≤40 mm in diameter) were split into two cohorts: those with no previous local treatment (Cohort A) or progressive brain metastases following prior local therapy (i.e., surgery, WBRT, or stereotactic radiosurgery [Cohort B]). Responses were found in both cohorts and in patients with either mutation. However, patients with V600K *BRAF*-mutant melanoma had a lower overall intracranial response rate compared to patients with tumors with the V600E *BRAF* mutation. In patients with V600E mutant tumors, the overall intracranial response (complete response + partial response) was 39.2% in Cohort A and 30.8% in Cohort B. For patients with V600K *BRAF*-mutation, the overall intracranial response rates were 6.7% and 22.2% in Cohorts A and B, respectively.[29] The decreased activity of dabrafenib in patients with V600K mutant melanoma brain metastases mirrored the lower extracranial response rates found in the phase II study of dabrafenib in patients with systemic melanoma and without brain metastases.[33]

Combined *BRAF* and *MEK* inhibition has resulted in better control of extracranial metastatic melanoma and improved survival in patients with *BRAF* V600E or V600K mutations.[34–36] Dabrafenib plus trametinib, as compared with dabrafenib or vemurafenib alone, significantly improves overall survival and progression-free survival in previously untreated patients with extracranial metastatic melanoma.[34,35] These studies did not recruit patients with untreated brain metastases. At present, there are at least two phase II trials investigating the efficacy of combination therapy in patients with *BRAF* V600E or V600K mutation-positive metastatic melanoma to the brain (NCT 01978236 and NCT 02039947).

Vemurafenib

Activity of vemurafenib for patients with melanoma brain metastases has been also reported in several cases with V600 *BRAF* mutation.[26–28,31,32] In one patient with solitary melanoma brain metastasis, neoadjuvant treatment with vemurafenib resulted in significant tumor necrosis and size reduction, making it amenable to surgical resection.[27] Also, a pilot study of 24 melanoma patients has suggested activity of vemurafenib in V600 *BRAF* mutant brain metastases, and a phase II trial of vemurafenib is ongoing (NCT01378975) and the results are anticipated shortly.

Immunotherapy

Interleukin-2

There are limited data on the safety and efficacy of high-dose interleukin-2 (IL-2) in untreated melanoma brain metastases.[37,38] Although a small, retrospective, single-institution study has reported complete response in 2 out of 15 patients with melanoma brain metastases, the results of a larger study by the U.S. National Cancer Institute showed limited activity, with overall response rate of 5.6% in patients with untreated brain metastases.[37,38] Given the intense nature of this treatment and lack of adequate data, IL-2's routine use in patients with melanoma brain metastases is not recommended.

Ipilimumab

Several case reports have shown the activity of ipilimumab in patients with melanoma brain metastases.[39–41] This has led to a phase II trial in which patients with melanoma brain metastases were divided in two cohorts based on symptoms and corticosteroid use.[42] Cohort A consisted of 51 patients with no neurological symptoms or corticosteroid use, while Cohort B included 23 patients who were symptomatic and on a stable dose of corticosteroids. Patients received one dose of 10 mg/kg intravenous ipilimumab every 3 weeks to a total of four doses (designated weeks 1, 4, 7, and 10; induction). Patients who were clinically stable at 24 weeks continued treatment with ipilimumab 10 mg/kg every 12 weeks (maintenance) until disease progression. CNS objective response rate after 12 weeks was 16% in Cohort A and 5% in Cohort B, respectively. After 12 weeks, CNS disease control (defined as complete response, partial response, or stable disease) was achieved in 25% of patients in Cohort A and 10% of patients in Cohort B.[42] Most importantly, the two-year survival rate for patients in Cohort A was similar to the two-year survival rate of patients without active brain metastases who were treated with ipilimumab in other studies. These data support the use of ipilimumab in asymptomatic patients with small melanoma brain metastases who do not require corticosteroids.[42]

These results have encouraged combination strategies using ipilimumab with other agents or treatment modalities. In a prospective cohort study, patients who had received ipilimumab in addition to definitive SRS had a longer median survival (21.3 months vs. 4.9 months) than patients who did not receive ipilimumab.[43]

The optimal dose of ipilimumab for the treatment of melanoma brain metastasis is yet to be determined. Although the dose of ipilimumab in the phase II trial conducted by Margolin et al. was 10 mg/kg, the clinical efficacy of ipilimumab at 3 mg/kg has been shown in several case reports.[39–42] In one patient treated with ipilimumab at a 3 mg/kg dose, pathological review of resected melanoma brain metastasis showed only cytotoxic anti-tumor immune responses, with little or no actively proliferating tumor. Therefore, while it remains to be proven in randomized phase III studies, we recommend using ipilimumab in patients with small melanoma brain metastases who do not require corticosteroids and can tolerate waiting two or three months for a response.

Nivolumab and Pembrolizumab

Nivolumab and pembrolizumab are fully human IgG4 programmed death 1 (PD-1) immune checkpoint inhibitors that selectively block the interaction of PD-1 with its two known ligands, PD-L1 and PD-L2.[44-46] Both antibodies have shown significant improvements in progression-free survival and overall survival in patients with metastatic melanoma.[44-46] However, their role in the treatment of patients with active brain metastases is not known, and studies are ongoing.

Leptomeningeal Metastases

Leptomeningeal metastases from melanoma commonly occur late in the course of disease and portend a grave prognosis. Median survival for patients with meningeal metastases from melanoma is about 10 weeks.[47] The common signs and symptoms include headache, nausea/vomiting, back or neck pain, sensory loss, and weakness.[47] In most cases, diagnosis can be made by MRI of the brain and/or spinal cord. However, lumbar puncture and analysis of cerebrospinal fluid are recommended to confirm the diagnosis and monitor response to treatment.

The main goal of treating leptomeningeal disease is palliative, with no standard of care to date. WBRT and spinal radiation therapy can be used in patients with symptomatic disease.

Variable responses have been associated with intrathecal chemotherapy alone or in combination with systemic chemotherapies such as temozolomide.[48,49]

Leptomeningeal metastases may respond to *BRAF* inhibitors. In two patients with tumors harboring V600 *BRAF* mutations, vemurafenib alone or with sequential WBRT resulted in marked response and long-term stabilization of leptomeningeal disease.[26,50] The role of immunotherapy in treatment of this condition is not clear. In one patient, WBRT followed with ipilimumab resulted in complete clinical and radiological response and survival of at least 1.5 years.[40]

Conclusion

The optimal management of melanoma brain metastases requires a multidisciplinary approach by neurosurgeons, radiation-oncologists, neuro-oncologists, and medical oncologists (Table 11.1). Aggressive local therapy with surgical resection or SRS should be considered in patients with limited intracranial

Table 11.1 Clinical Trials in Patients with Melanoma Brain Metastases

Study	Design	Tumor Type	Therapy	N	Median OS (mos)	HR	CNS-ORR
Surgical Resection							
Fife et al. [3]	Retrospective	Melanoma	Surgery	47	8.7*	0.436*	
			WBRT	236	3.4	0.851	
			Supportive care	210	2.1		
Sampson et al. [7]	Retrospective	Melanoma	Surgery	52	6.5*		
			WBRT	180	4		
Noordijk et al. [8]	Randomized	Solid tumors, including melanoma	Surgery + WBRT	32	10*		
			WBRT	31	6		
WBRT post-surgical resection							
Fife et al. [3]	Retrospective	Melanoma	Surgery + WBRT	158	8.9		
			Surgery	47	8.7		
Sampson et al. [7]	Retrospective	Melanoma	Surgery	52	6.5		
			Surgery + WBRT	87	8.9		
SRS							
Radbill et al. [13]	Retrospective	Melanoma	SRS alone	32	6.5		
Chemotherapy							
Agarwala et al. [24]	Single-arm Phase II	Melanoma	Temozolomide	151	3.2		6%
Avril et al. [23]	Randomized Phase III	Melanoma	Fotemustine	22			5.9%
			Dacarbazine	21			0%

(continued)

Table 11.1 Continued

Study	Design	Tumor Type	Therapy	N	Median OS (mos)	HR	CNS-ORR
BRAF Inhibitors							
Long et al.[29]	Single-arm Phase II	BRAF-mutant melanoma	Dabrafenib	172	16.3–33.1		30.8–39.2%
Interleukin-2							
Guirguis et al.[37]	Retrospective	Melanoma or renal cell carcinoma	Interleukin-2	64			5.6–18.5%
Ipilimumab							
Margolin et al.[42]	Single-arm Phase II	Melanoma	Ipilimumab	72	3.7–7		5–16%

*Statistically significant

N = Number of patients; OS = Overall survival; HR = Hazard ratio; CNS-ORR = Central nervous system overall response rate; WBRT = Whole-brain radiotherapy; SRS = Stereotactic radiosurgery disease, controlled extracranial disease, and a favorable prognosis. In patients who undergo local therapy, the addition of WRBT should be considered carefully since there is increased treatment-related toxicity and no improvement in overall survival. Hence, the detrimental effect of WBRT on quality of life and cognitive abilities should be considered before using this treatment modality.

In symptomatic patients with multiple intracranial metastases who are deemed ineligible for aggressive local therapy, WRBT may be used to alleviate the symptoms.

Conventional cytotoxic chemotherapeutic agents have limited activity against melanoma brain metastases, and their use is not recommended. Encouraging results have been observed with the use of dabrafenib and vemurafenib in patients with V600 *BRAF* mutant melanoma brain metastases. Ipilimumab has shown activity and survival benefit in patients with asymptomatic melanoma brain metastases who do not require corticosteroids. However, with the advent of new targeted and immunotherapies, it is imperative to encourage the enrollment of patients with melanoma brain metastasis to clinical trials testing new targeted therapies and combination strategies.

References

1. Barnholtz-Sloan JS, Sloan AE, Davis FG, Vigneau FD, Lai P, Sawaya RE. Incidence proportions of brain metastases in patients diagnosed (1973 to 2001) in the Metropolitan Detroit Cancer Surveillance System. *J Clin Oncol.* 2004;22(14):2865–2872.

2. Davies MA, Liu P, McIntyre S, et al. Prognostic factors for survival in melanoma patients with brain metastases. *Cancer.* 2011;117(8):1687–1696.

3. Fife KM, Colman MH, Stevens GN, et al. Determinants of outcome in melanoma patients with cerebral metastases. *J Clin Oncol.* 2004;22(7):1293–1300.

4. Staudt M, Lasithiotakis K, Leiter U, et al. Determinants of survival in patients with brain metastases from cutaneous melanoma. *Br J Cancer.* 2010;102(8):1213–1218.

5. Sperduto PW, Kased N, Roberge D, et al. Summary report on the graded prognostic assessment: an accurate and facile diagnosis-specific tool to estimate survival for patients with brain metastases. *J Clin Oncol.* 2012;30(4):419–425.

6. Eigentler TK, Figl A, Krex D, et al. Number of metastases, serum lactate dehydrogenase level, and type of treatment are prognostic factors in patients with brain metastases of malignant melanoma. *Cancer.* 2011;117(8):1697–1703.

7. Sampson JH, Carter JH Jr, Friedman AH, Seigler HF. Demographics, prognosis, and therapy in 702 patients with brain metastases from malignant melanoma. *J Neurosurg.* 1998;88(1):11–20.

8. Noordijk EM, Vecht CJ, Haaxma-Reiche H, et al. The choice of treatment of single brain metastasis should be based on extracranial tumor activity and age. *Int J Radiat Oncol Biol Phys.* 1994;29(4):711–717.

9. Margolin K, Atkins B, Thompson A, et al. Temozolomide and whole brain irradiation in melanoma metastatic to the brain: a phase II trial of the Cytokine Working Group. *J Cancer Res Clin Oncol.* 2002;128(4):214–218.

10. Skeie BS, Skeie GO, Enger PO, et al. Gamma knife surgery in brain melanomas: absence of extracranial metastases and tumor volume strongest

indicators of prolonged survival. *World Neurosurg.* 2011;75(5–6):684–691; discussion, 598–603.

11. Mornex F, Thomas L, Mohr P, et al. A prospective randomized multicentre phase III trial of fotemustine plus whole brain irradiation versus fotemustine alone in cerebral metastases of malignant melanoma. *Melanoma Res.* 2003;13(1):97–103.

12. Atkins MB, Sosman JA, Agarwala S, et al. Temozolomide, thalidomide, and whole brain radiation therapy for patients with brain metastasis from metastatic melanoma: a phase II Cytokine Working Group study. *Cancer.* 2008;113(8):2139–2145.

13. Radbill AE, Fiveash JF, Falkenberg ET, et al. Initial treatment of melanoma brain metastases using gamma knife radiosurgery: an evaluation of efficacy and toxicity. *Cancer.* 2004;101(4):825–833.

14. Lavine SD, Petrovich Z, Cohen-Gadol AA, et al. Gamma knife radiosurgery for metastatic melanoma: an analysis of survival, outcome, and complications. *Neurosurgery.* 1999;44(1):59–64; discussion, 64–56.

15. Liew DN, Kano H, Kondziolka D, et al. Outcome predictors of gamma knife surgery for melanoma brain metastases. Clinical article. *J Neurosurg.* 2011;114(3):769–779.

16. Chang EL, Selek U, Hassenbusch SJ 3rd, et al. Outcome variation among "radioresistant" brain metastases treated with stereotactic radiosurgery. *Neurosurgery.* 2005;56(5):936–945; discussion, 936–945.

17. Soltys SG, Adler JR, Lipani JD, et al. Stereotactic radiosurgery of the postoperative resection cavity for brain metastases. *Int J Radiat Oncol Biol Phys.* 2008;70(1):187–193.

18. Jensen CA, Chan MD, McCoy TP, et al. Cavity-directed radiosurgery as adjuvant therapy after resection of a brain metastasis. *J Neurosurg.* 2011;114(6):1585–1591.

19. Choi CY, Chang SD, Gibbs IC, et al. Stereotactic radiosurgery of the postoperative resection cavity for brain metastases: prospective evaluation of target margin on tumor control. *Int J Radiat Oncol Biol Phys.* 2012;84(2):336–342.

20. Kocher M, Soffietti R, Abacioglu U, et al. Adjuvant whole-brain radiotherapy versus observation after radiosurgery or surgical resection of one to three cerebral metastases: results of the EORTC 22952-26001 study. *J Clin Oncol.* 2011;29(2):134–141.

21. Aoyama H, Shirato H, Tago M, et al. Stereotactic radiosurgery plus whole-brain radiation therapy vs stereotactic radiosurgery alone for treatment of brain metastases: a randomized controlled trial. *JAMA.* 2006;295(21):2483–2491.

22. Chang EL, Wefel JS, Hess KR, et al. Neurocognition in patients with brain metastases treated with radiosurgery or radiosurgery plus whole-brain irradiation: a randomised controlled trial. *Lancet Oncol.* 2009;10(11):1037–1044.

23. Avril MF, Aamdal S, Grob JJ, et al. Fotemustine compared with dacarbazine in patients with disseminated malignant melanoma: a phase III study. *J Clin Oncol.* 2004;22(6):1118–1125.

24. Agarwala SS, Kirkwood JM, Gore M, et al. Temozolomide for the treatment of brain metastases associated with metastatic melanoma: a phase II study. *J Clin Oncol.* 2004;22(11):2101–2107.

25. Jakob JA, Bassett RL, Jr., Ng CS, et al. NRAS mutation status is an independent prognostic factor in metastatic melanoma. *Cancer.* 2012;118(16):4014–4023.

26. Schafer N, Scheffler B, Stuplich M, et al. Vemurafenib for leptomeningeal melanomatosis. *J Clin Oncol.* 2013;31(11):e173–174.

27. Kolar GR, Miller-Thomas MM, Schmidt RE, Simpson JR, Rich KM, Linette GP. Neoadjuvant treatment of a solitary melanoma brain metastasis with vemurafenib. *J Clin Oncol.* 2013;31(3):e40–e43.

28. Rochet NM, Kottschade LA, Markovic SN. Vemurafenib for melanoma metastases to the brain. *N Engl J Med.* 2011;365(25):2439–2441.

29. Long GV, Trefzer U, Davies MA, et al. Dabrafenib in patients with Val600Glu or Val600Lys *BRAF*-mutant melanoma metastatic to the brain (BREAK-MB): a multicentre, open-label, phase 2 trial. *Lancet Oncol.* 2012;13(11):1087–1095.

30. Falchook GS, Long GV, Kurzrock R, et al. Dabrafenib in patients with melanoma, untreated brain metastases, and other solid tumours: a phase 1 dose-escalation trial. *Lancet.* 2012;379(9829):1893–1901.

31. van den Brom RR, de Vries EG, Schroder CP, Hospers GA. Effect of vemurafenib on a V600R melanoma brain metastasis. *Eur J Cancer.* 2013;49(7):1795–1796.

32. Klein O, Clements A, Menzies AM, O'Toole S, Kefford RF, Long GV. *BRAF* inhibitor activity in V600R metastatic melanoma. *Eur J Cancer.* 2013;49(5):1073–1079.

33. Ascierto PA, Minor D, Ribas A, et al. Phase II trial (BREAK-2) of the *BRAF* inhibitor dabrafenib (GSK2118436) in patients with metastatic melanoma. *J Clin Oncol.* 2013;31(26):3205–3211.

34. Robert C, Karaszewska B, Schachter J, et al. Improved overall survival in melanoma with combined dabrafenib and trametinib. *N Engl J Med.* 2015;372(1):30–39.

35. Long GV, Stroyakovskiy D, Gogas H, et al. Combined *BRAF* and *MEK* inhibition versus *BRAF* inhibition alone in melanoma. *N Engl J Med.* 2014;371(20):1877–1888.

36. Johnson DB, Flaherty KT, Weber JS, et al. Combined *BRAF* (dabrafenib) and *MEK* inhibition (trametinib) in patients with *BRAFV600*-mutant melanoma experiencing progression with single-agent *BRAF* inhibitor. *J Clin Oncol.* 2014;32(33):3697–3704.

37. Guirguis LM, Yang JC, White DE, et al. Safety and efficacy of high-dose interleukin-2 therapy in patients with brain metastases. *J Immunother.* 2002;25(1):82–87.

38. Powell S, Dudek AZ. Single-institution outcome of high-dose interleukin-2 (HD IL-2) therapy for metastatic melanoma and analysis of favorable response in brain metastases. *Anticancer Res.* 2009;29(10):4189–4193.

39. Hodi FS, Oble DA, Drappatz J, et al. CTLA-4 blockade with ipilimumab induces significant clinical benefit in a female with melanoma metastases to the CNS. *Nat Clin Pract. Oncol.* 2008;5(9):557–561.

40. Bot I, Blank CU, Brandsma D. Clinical and radiological response of leptomeningeal melanoma after whole brain radiotherapy and ipilimumab. *J Neurol.* 2012;259(9):1976–1978.

41. Schartz NE, Farges C, Madelaine I, et al. Complete regression of a previously untreated melanoma brain metastasis with ipilimumab. *Melanoma Res.* 2010;20(3):247–250.

42. Margolin K, Ernstoff MS, Hamid O, et al. Ipilimumab in patients with melanoma and brain metastases: an open-label, phase 2 trial. *Lancet Oncol.* 2012;13(5):459–465.

43. Knisely JP, Yu JB, Flanigan J, Sznol M, Kluger HM, Chiang VL. Radiosurgery for melanoma brain metastases in the ipilimumab era and the possibility of longer survival. *J Neurosurg.* 2012;117(2):227–233.

44. Topalian SL, Sznol M, McDermott DF, et al. Survival, durable tumor remission, and long-term safety in patients with advanced melanoma receiving nivolumab. *J Clin Oncol.* 2014;32(10):1020–1030.

45. Robert C, Long GV, Brady B, et al. Nivolumab in previously untreated melanoma without *BRAF* mutation. *N Engl J Med.* 2015;372(4):320–330.

46. Robert C, Ribas A, Wolchok JD, et al. Anti-programmed-death-receptor-1 treatment with pembrolizumab in ipilimumab-refractory advanced melanoma: a randomised dose-comparison cohort of a phase 1 trial. *Lancet.* 2014; 384(9948):1109–1117.

47. Harstad L, Hess KR, Groves MD. Prognostic factors and outcomes in patients with leptomeningeal melanomatosis. *Neuro-oncology.* 2008;10(6):1010–1018.

48. Schaefer N, Rasch K, Moehlenbruch M, et al. Leptomeningeal melanomatosis: stabilization of disease due to radiation, temozolomide and intrathecal liposomal cytarabine. *Acta Oncol.* 2011;50(8):1260–1262.

49. Pape E, Desmedt E, Zairi F, et al. Leptomeningeal metastasis in melanoma: a prospective clinical study of nine patients. *In Vivo.* 2012;26(6):1079–1086.

50. Lee JM, Mehta UN, Dsouza LH, Guadagnolo BA, Sanders DL, Kim KB. Long-term stabilization of leptomeningeal disease with whole-brain radiation therapy in a patient with metastatic melanoma treated with vemurafenib: a case report. *Melanoma Res.* 2013;23(2):175–178.

Chapter 12

Management of Mucosal and Ocular Melanoma

Alexander N. Shoushtari and Richard D. Carvajal

Malignant melanomas represent 1–2% of all malignancies, with the vast majority of cases being cutaneous primary tumors. In 5–10% of cases, however, melanoma arises from mucosal areas, the uveal tract of the eye, or an unknown primary site. Recently, advances in targeted kinase inhibitors and immune therapy have revolutionized the treatment of melanoma. These trials were largely conducted in cutaneous melanoma (CM), however, and there are fewer published data regarding therapy in mucosal and ocular melanomas. Given the increasing knowledge of the distinct molecular changes underlying these various melanoma subtypes, it is increasingly important to understand the distinct epidemiology, presentation, prognosis, and treatment options for these subtypes.

Mucosal Melanoma

Background, Epidemiology, and Molecular Alterations

The incidence of mucosal melanoma (MM) in the United States is approximately 1.5 cases per million.[1] The percentage of melanoma cases that are MMs varies by ethnicity, from less than 2% in Caucasians to 10% in African-Americans and nearly one-third in Chinese patients.[1,2] The most common site of MM is the head and neck region (55% of cases), followed by anorectal (24%), vulvovaginal (18%), and urinary tract (3%).[1] There is a female predominance of 1.5–2:1, which is largely due to a higher rate of vulvovaginal melanomas compared to penile melanomas.[1] MM typically affects patients in their seventh decade of life, approximately a decade older than patients with CM.

Most head and neck mucosal melanomas (HNMM) arise in the nasal cavity (49%), paranasal sinuses (23%), or oral cavity (19%). Less commonly, the nasopharynx (5%), oropharynx (3%), larynx, and esophagus (<1%) are implicated as primary sites.[3] Nasal cavity melanomas typically present with epistaxis or nasal obstruction, while oropharyngeal lesions are most often found on dental examination or with bleeding or ill-fitting dentures.[4]

Anorectal melanomas (AMMs) represent between 1–5% of all cancers of the anal canal.[1] Published reports estimate between two-thirds and 90% arise near the dentate line, although due to the large size of most of these lesions at the time of diagnosis, a precise location is not always possible.[5,6] As a result of its rarity and inconspicuous anatomical location, AMMs are, in general, larger and more deeply invasive than cutaneous lesions at diagnosis.[7]

Vulvovaginal melanomas (VVMs) represent the majority of melanomas in the genitourinary tract. In females, the majority of VVMs are pigmented lesions of the vulva; lesions of the lower third of the vagina and the cervix are rarer. Together, melanomas represent 10% of all vulvar cancers.[8] Median age of diagnosis in most studies is in the mid-50s to early 60s, although children have been reported with VVM.

A landmark study by Curtin et al. quantified the prevalence of activating mutations in BRAF, a member of the mitogen-activated protein kinase (MAPK) pathway, and NRAS, a Ras family member that activates both MAPK and PI3K signaling pathways, in four groups of melanomas: mucosal melanomas ($n = 20$), acral melanomas ($n = 36$), and cutaneous melanomas with ($n = 30$) and without ($n = 40$) evidence of chronic sun-induced damage.[9] In contrast to cutaneous melanomas, mucosal melanomas had much lower rates of mutation: BRAF in 11% and NRAS in 5%.[9] Specific mucosal melanoma subtypes may have higher rates of NRAS mutations. One series found 6 out of 16 cases of esophageal melanoma had an NRAS mutation,[10] whereas another series in vaginal melanoma identified 3 out of 7 cases with this mutation.[11]

Further genetic analysis of 102 mucosal melanomas that were wild-type for BRAF and NRAS identified 39% that had mutations or amplifications in KIT (also known as CD117), a Type III receptor tyrosine kinase that activates MAPK and PI3K signaling.[12] Notably, these mutations lie in codons distinct from those found in gastrointestinal stromal tumors. Follow-up case series confirmed similar mutation (15–38%) and amplification (20–33%) rates.[13–16] Interestingly, a case series of 167 Chinese mucosal melanomas found lower mutation and amplification rates of 10% each,[2] suggesting regional variation in underlying molecular alterations. These alterations have important therapeutic implications, as will be discussed below.

Workup and Staging of Mucosal Melanomas

Mucosal melanoma subtypes vary in their clinical behavior and staging classifications. A nasopharyngeal endoscopic evaluation by an experienced practitioner is mandatory for HNMM to assess for multifocal primary disease. For AMM and VVM, careful examination of the primary sites (e.g., involvement of sphincter) and the superficial inguinal lymph node basin may give prognostic information and guide treatment. For all subtypes, computed tomography (CT) of the chest, abdomen, and pelvis with contrast is recommended. CT of the neck may be helpful to identify lymph node (LN) metastases for HNMM, and endorectal magnetic resonance imaging (MRI) may help define sphincter involvement for AMMs. The use of sentinel LN mapping and biopsy is feasible; however, the clinical implications of sentinel lymph node involvement in mucosal melanoma are not clear.

In contrast to cutaneous melanoma, there is currently no universally accepted staging system for mucosal melanomas. Due to its ease of use and generalizability, a reasonable system is one proposed by Ballantyne in 1970.[17]

It describes three stages: localized tumor, regional lymph node spread, and distant metastases. One of the limitations of the Ballantyne system, however, is the fact that the vast majority of patients present with localized, Ballantyne Stage I disease, but many will subsequently develop metastases.[18] AMMs are most commonly staged using this system. HNMM has a specific classification in the American Joint Committee on Cancer (AJCC) 7th edition, where the least advanced tumors are classified as stage III, reflecting their poor overall prognosis.[19] For VVMs, staging system varies by subtype. Vulvar lesions can be classified using the AJCC 7th edition for cutaneous melanoma, while vaginal lesions are classified using the Ballantyne system.[20]

Prognostic Factors

Overall, patients with mucosal melanomas have a poorer prognosis than their cutaneous counterparts.[7,21,22] There is much heterogeneity, however, in clinical behavior and prognostic factors. For example, within HNMMs, 25% of oral cavity tumors presented with LN metastases, versus only 6% of sinonasal primaries.[23] There is no consistent evidence that LN disease affects prognosis, probably due to the ability to surgically salvage this region. Local recurrence occurs in up to 80% of cases and predicts poor outcomes, with salvage rates generally less than 25%.[18,22] AMMs have an equal rate of regional and distant spread at presentation of 20%. Median survival with local, regional, and distant disease is estimated at 24, 17, and 8 months, respectively.[24] For VVMs, vulvar primaries have a better prognosis than vaginal or cervical primaries. Five-year overall survival rates for vulvar lesions are reported to be up to 55% in some series, versus generally less than 25% for vaginal primaries.[25] For specific clinicopathological features linked with prognosis in each subtype, see Table 12.1.

Locoregional Therapy

Surgical resection is the cornerstone of curative therapy, regardless of mucosal melanoma subtype. For HNMM, local recurrences are common, and multiple resections may be necessary to obtain negative margins. Oral cavity tumors often utilize sentinel LN evaluation due to the higher risk of regional spread from this site. Adjuvant radiation therapy has been shown to decrease locoregional recurrence rates but does not improve OS.[26]

The surgical plan for AMMs varies, depending on sphincter involvement. Gross sphincter involvement necessitates an abdominoperineal resection (APR). Other cases may utilize a wide local excision (WLE) and spare sphincter control. Although prospective comparison is lacking, mounting evidence suggests APR improves only local control and not overall survival (OS).[27] As a result, many melanoma referral centers such as Memorial Sloan-Kettering Cancer Center favor WLE, with APR utilized as salvage upon recurrence. Similar retrospective data in VVM support the use of WLE over pelvic exenteration or vulvectomy.[28] Sentinel LN excision is feasible in these disease types, but its role has yet to be validated, given that the risk of mortality is strongly linked to development of distant metastatic disease.[27,28]

Adjuvant radiation therapy (RT) is utilized at many referral centers to increase local control rates, especially for HNMM.[29–31] For AMM, an updated

Table 12.1 Clinical and Prognostic Variability of Mucosal Melanoma Subtypes

Subtype	M:F	Most Common Location	Presenting Symptom	Poor Prognostic Factors*	Suggested Staging System	5-Year Survival
Head and Neck	1:1	Nasal cavity	Epistaxis, obstruction, dental abnormality	Age >70, depth, (+) margins, recurrence, distant mets, LVI, # mitoses	AJCC 7, Head and neck	30–35%
Anorectal	2:3	Anal canal	Hemato-chezia, mass, pain	Age, male sex, size, depth, ulceration, perineural invasion	Ballantyne	10–20%
Vulvovaginal (Genito-urinary)	1:10	Vulva	Mass, pain, bleeding	Non-vulvar 1°; Breslow depth; (+) nodes	*Vulvar:* AJCC 7 Cutaneous *Non-Vulvar:* Ballantyne	*Vulvar:* 30–55% *Non-Vulvar:* 5–25%

*Reflect general trends in prognosis when multiple case series conflict on prognostic variables.
AJCC 7 = American Joint Committee on Cancer 7th Edition; LVI = lymphovascular invasion

case series from MD Anderson reports local and regional control rates following WLE plus RT of 82–88%.[32] Due to high rates of distant metastases, adjuvant RT does not improve overall survival.[24,27–33] Its role in VVM is not well defined.

Systemic Therapy

The role of systemic therapy for mucosal melanoma in the adjuvant setting is unclear, and there is no current standard of care. The only prospective trial of adjuvant therapy was performed in 189 Chinese patients with resected AJCC stage II/III mucosal melanoma who were randomized to either expectant observation, high-dose interferon alpha (IFNα), or cisplatin plus temozolomide.[34] This study reported an increase in recurrence-free survival (RFS) from 5.4 to 9.4 and 20.8 months with the addition of IFNα and chemotherapy, respectively. The estimated OS of these three groups was 21.2 months versus 40.4 months and 48.7 months, respectively.[34] Given the emerging evidence of genetic differences between Asian and Caucasian mucosal melanomas (see above), this striking result may reflect a different underlying biology of disease. Nonetheless, this study provides a rationale for offering adjuvant temozolomide and cisplatin to select patients with good performance status and few comorbidities. This study should be replicated before adjuvant chemotherapy is considered standard of care.

For metastatic mucosal melanoma, no systemic therapy has been shown to improve progression-free survival (PFS) or OS. Recent advances in treating metastatic cutaneous melanoma with immune-activating agents such as ipilimumab[35,36] have led to their use in patients with MM. Two retrospective series have been reported looking at the efficacy of ipilimumab, specifically in mucosal melanoma.[37,38] They both demonstrated a relatively low response rate (7–12% by immune-related response criteria) and a median OS of 6.4 months.[37,38] As in CMs, however, durable responses were described, suggesting a subset of patients benefits due to unknown underlying differences in tumor or systemic immunophenotype. Future prospective trials of immune-activating therapy in MM are warranted.

The knowledge that mucosal melanomas harbor alterations in *KIT* and, to a lesser extent, *BRAF* and *NRAS* signaling, has therapeutic significance. Imatinib has been utilized in three recent trials that selected for *KIT* mutant melanomas. In one phase II study, 28 patients of varying melanoma subtypes were treated with imatinib 400 mg twice daily, and durable responses were seen in four patients, including two with complete responses that lasted over 90 weeks.[39] A second study confirmed that patients with *KIT* mutant MMs who responded to imatinib had significantly increased median PFS and OS.[40] A third study identified 77% of *KIT* mutant patients who responded to imatinib.[41] In all three studies, patients who benefitted were more likely to have mutations in exons 11 or 13 rather than exon 17 or *KIT* amplifications.

Tumors from patients with mucosal melanomas should be studied for alterations in *KIT, BRAF,* and *NRAS.* Providers should discuss with their patients whether a referral to a tertiary melanoma center is feasible, to facilitate genetic analysis and/or participation in clinical trials that may expand their options for systemic therapy.

Uveal Melanoma

Epidemiology

Uveal melanoma (UM) arises from melanocytes of the iris, ciliary body, and choroid, which together comprise the uveal tract of the eye. UM is the most common primary intraocular malignancy in adults, accounting for 5% of all melanoma diagnoses each year. The yearly incidence is 5–6 cases per million, and it is more common in males, with a M:F ratio of 1.2:1. The median age at diagnosis is 62 years, and Caucasians are approximately 98% of all reported cases.[42]

Staging and Prognosis

Distant metastases occur in approximately 50% of patients within 20 years of initial diagnosis. The liver is the most common site of metastasis, representing the initial site for 60% of patients and eventually affecting over 90%.[43,44] Other common sites of metastasis include the lung, soft tissue, bone, and brain.[43] Due largely to the historical lack of efficacious systemic treatment strategies, the prognosis of metastatic disease is dismal. Median OS ranges from 6–12 months.[45,46]

Clinical predictors of worse disease outcome include age over 60, the presence of hepatic metastases (versus lung or soft tissue), and shorter intervals from diagnosis to metastasis.[43] Clinical features of the primary tumor that predict poorer outcomes include larger tumor diameter, thickness, and location in the ciliary body versus the rest of uveal tract.[47]

In the *AJCC 7th Edition Cancer Staging Manual*, stages I–III are predicted by tumor diameter and thickness as well as degree of ciliary body or extraocular involvement. Any spread to lymph node and other organs is considered stage IV disease. In a large retrospective analysis of 7,731 patients, this system stratified for risk of metastasis and death. For example, T1 through T4 tumors had 10-year risk of death of 8%, 13%, 27%, and 43%, respectively.[48]

In the early 1990s, the genetic basis of these clinical factors began to be elucidated. Cytogenetic studies discerned that UM with monosomy 3 or duplication of 8q24 had a 50% rate of metastasis at three years, and had worse disease-free survival (DFS) and OS.[49,50] Another method of stratification came with gene expression profiling (GEP). The current assay is a 15-gene GEP panel (DecisionDx-UM, Castle Biosciences) that stratifies tumors into low metastatic potential (Class 1) and high metastatic potential (Class 2) groups. The four-year risk of metastasis in low-risk tumors was <5%, versus >80% in high-risk tumors.[51] This assay was prospectively validated in 459 patients and, in this series, was superior to both Tumor Node Metastasis (TNM) and monosomy 3 risk-classification strategies.[51] Their genetic background and impact on management are summarized in Table 12.2.

Surveillance

Given the high rate of metastatic disease, particularly for patients with high-risk tumors, many centers advocate for routine surveillance. Although surveillance has not proven to improve survival, it may have other advantages. Generally, suggested regimens include hepatic function panels, which have good negative predictive values in some series, and cross-sectional imaging. Imaging modalities include CT of chest, abdomen, and pelvis; MRI of abdomen and pelvis; abdominal ultrasound, or positron emission tomography (PET). Each modality has relative strengths and weaknesses.[52] Although ultrasound is inexpensive and spares radiation, it is operator-dependent and insensitive, especially in more obese patients. While CT scans are widely available and represent a relatively uniform way to screen the whole body, they have a low

Table 12.2 Comparison of Low-Risk, Class I, and High-Risk, Class II Subgroups of Uveal Melanoma

	Low Risk	**High Risk**
GEP Classification	Class I	Class II
Metastasis Risk at 4 Years	<5%	>80%
Recommended Surveillance	No specific surveillance	LFTs, CT/MRI every 3–6 months
Chromosomal Abnormalities	Disomy 3 Disomy 8	3p loss; 8q24 amplification
Associated Genetic Alterations	*SF3B1* mutation	BAP1 loss MYC amplification
GEP = gene expression profile; LFT = liver function test		

positive predictive value. While PET/CT are universally positive in cutaneous melanomas, a recent study suggests uveal melanoma metastases are positive only 40% of the time and, in other studies, PET/CT is insensitive for liver metastases less than 1 cm in size.[53] MRI may be more sensitive for hepatic metastases. As a result, many referral centers favor screening with MR of the liver, with or without imaging of the chest and pelvis, every 3–12 months, with the interval selected based upon estimated risk of recurrence, with the goal of detecting asymptomatic, oligometastatic disease.[52] The optimal overall duration of surveillance is unknown, and it may be reasonable to decrease the frequency of imaging to annual imaging 5–10 years after diagnosis.

Treatment of Uveal Melanoma

Local Therapy

Historically, enucleation has been the primary treatment for uveal melanomas. In an effort to spare the globe in these patients, radiation therapy (RT) has been increasingly utilized, with retrospective studies reporting equivalent rates of local control, metastasis, and OS for medium-sized melanomas.[54–56] The two broad categories of RT utilize either proton beam or brachytherapy with plaque insertion. The only randomized, phase III trial (Collaborative Ocular Melanoma Study [COMS]) comparing enucleation with RT utilized plaque iodine-125 therapy in medium-sized tumors (apical height 2.5–10 mm or basal diameter ≥16 mm). It demonstrated no difference in overall survival at 5 and 12 years.[57,58] A randomized COMS trial reported no mortality benefit with combined neoadjuvant RT and enucleation for large tumors.[59]

Overall, local therapy choices are guided by the size of the primary tumor; its location relative to the macula, optic disk, or anterior segment; and comorbidities such visual status of the fellow eye or systemic vasculopathies. Despite improvements in RT and surgical techniques, the rates of distant metastases and disease-specific mortality remain unchanged.[60]

Locoregional Treatments

Since the vast majority of patients with metastatic UM die of sequelae of hepatic metastases, various treatment strategies have been attempted to treat this regional site of disease. A prospective trial from France utilized multimodality surgical and hepatic-directed multiagent chemotherapy for UM patients with hepatic metastases. For the minority of patients for whom a complete surgical resection was possible, overall survival was increased from a median of 9 months to 22 months.[61]

Landmark physiological studies have established that, while the normal liver is perfused by both arterial and portal systems, neoplasms are disproportionately fed by the arterial system.[62–64] As a result, multiple techniques utilizing arterial catheterization have been utilized, such as hepatic transarterial chemoembolization (TACE), which combines a liver-directed chemotherapy agent such as cisplatin with the ischemic effects of embolization. Multiple studies have demonstrated partial responses in a substantial minority of patients; unfortunately, there is generally no improvement in OS.[65] There have been no randomized studies of TACE to support its routine use, but selected cases with low disease burden may derive benefit.[65]

The first phase III trial utilizing locoregional therapy, a percutaneous hepatic perfusion trial of melphalan, reported 93 patients who were randomized to receive 4–6 treatments with melphalan versus observation.[66] While it met its primary endpoint of increasing median hepatic PFS from 49 days to 245 days, no overall survival benefit was observed, and this therapy failed to achieve regulatory approval. A randomized phase III trial of fotemustine administered via hepatic artery infusion versus intravenously demonstrated a response rate of 11% versus 2%, but, again, there was no difference in OS.[67]

Systemic Treatments

Conventional cytotoxic chemotherapy has been ineffective in metastatic UM. A phase II study of temozolomide (TMZ) reported no objective responses and an OS of 6.7 months.[46] A retrospective review of 143 patients with metastatic UM treated at MD Anderson noted one objective response.[68] Eleven prospective trials have treated 422 patients with systemic chemotherapy, and the objective response rate ranged from 0–6%.[46,67,69–77] The immune checkpoint activator ipilimumab is approved for metastatic cutaneous melanoma, but data in uveal melanoma are limited. Multiple retrospective analyses of heavily pretreated cohorts indicate clinical benefit for a subset of patients,[78–81] with the largest series of 83 patients demonstrating 3-month stable disease rate of 35%.[81] Further study is needed to define the role of immune-activating agents in uveal melanoma.

Genomic Alterations and Impact on Systemic Therapy

Recent advances in our understanding of the underlying genetic alterations of UM have provided potential novel therapeutic strategies. The most critical insight thus far into mechanisms of UM tumor growth came in 2009–2010, when van Raamsdonk and colleagues reported two mutually exclusive activating mutations in G-alpha subunits (*GNAQ* and *GNA11*) of UM cells that resulted in constitutive signaling downstream of G-protein coupled receptors.[82,83] As a result, several downstream growth signaling pathways are up-regulated, including mitogen activated protein kinase (MAPK), protein kinase C (PKC), and phosphidylinositol-3 kinase (PI3K)/mammalian Target of Rapamycin (mTOR)/Akt.[84] This discovery has played a major role in accelerating the rational development of novel therapeutic strategies in uveal melanoma.

A randomized phase II trial of the MEK inhibitor selumetinib versus chemotherapy with either temozolomide or dacarbazine (investigator's choice) was the first to demonstrate clinical benefit in metastatic UM. PFS increased from 7 weeks with chemotherapy to 16 weeks with selumetinib.[85] Downstream effectors of the MAPK pathway were down-regulated, suggesting adequate target inhibition, and radiological response was significantly correlated with pERK inhibition. Interestingly, there was no significant difference in the degree of PFS benefit from selumetinib among the prespecified subset of patients with exon 5 mutations in *GNAQ* or *GNA11* ($n = 83$ of 98 total) versus those wild-type in exon 5 ($n = 15$). This lack of difference in PFS may be due to the high prevalence of exon 4 mutations in the "wild-type" cohort that activate similar signaling cascades.[83] In this trial, only 5/15 samples of wild-type for exon 5 had adequate specimen available for exon 4 testing, and 3/5 were mutant.[85]

Based on the promise of this randomized phase II trial, a randomized phase III trial comparing dacarbazine alone with dacarbazine plus selumetinib has completed accrual, and results are expected by late 2015 (NCT01974752). If these results are positive, selumetinib could be the first agent approved specifically for advanced uveal melanoma. Other clinical trials are now underway targeting other pathways such as PKC and PI3K/Akt, either alone or in combination with MEK inhibition.

Given the numerous recent advances in the treatment of metastatic cutaneous melanomas, the question arises: Should a patient with newly diagnosed metastatic uveal melanoma be treated with CTLA-4 and PD-1 inhibitors or on uveal melanoma clinical trials? Given the promising PFS data for MEK inhibition and the lack of prospective data for immune-activating agents in uveal melanoma, we consider participation in a clinical trial the most appropriate front-line therapy. Furthermore, there is emerging evidence that ipilimumab has greatest efficacy in melanomas with higher mutational burdens that create antigenic "neoepitopes."[86] As a result, ipilimumab may not be the ideal agent for treating uveal melanomas, which have much lower mutational burdens.[87]

Conclusion

The relative rarity of noncutaneous melanomas has historically impeded progress in our understanding of the epidemiology, biology, and clinical behavior of these diseases. Over the past several years, however, it has become clear that melanomas arising from mucosal surfaces and the uveal tract are biologically distinct from cutaneous melanomas. Mucosal and uveal melanomas harbor distinct mutational patterns compared to cutaneous melanomas that may underlie their distinct responses to kinase inhibitors as well as to cytotoxic and immunological agents. Given our increasing understanding of relevant molecular targets for each subtype of melanoma, future clinical trials promise to improve our ability to treat patients with these tumors.

References

1. Chang AE, Karnell LH, Menck HR. The National Cancer Data Base report on cutaneous and noncutaneous melanoma: a summary of 84,836 cases from the past decade. The American College of Surgeons Commission on Cancer and the American Cancer Society. *Cancer*. Oct 15, 1998;83(8):1664–1678.

2. Kong Y, Si L, Zhu Y, et al. Large-scale analysis of *KIT* aberrations in Chinese patients with melanoma. *Clin Cancer Res*. Apr 1, 2011;17(7):1684–1691.

3. Jethanamest D, Vila PM, Sikora AG, Morris LG. Predictors of survival in mucosal melanoma of the head and neck. *Ann Surg Oncol*. Oct 2011;18(10):2748–2756.

4. Gavriel H, McArthur G, Sizeland A, Henderson M. Review: mucosal melanoma of the head and neck. *Melanoma Res*. Aug 2011;21(4):257–266.

5. Baskies AM, Sugarbaker EV, Chretien PB, Deckers PJ. Anorectal melanoma. The role of posterior pelvic exenteration. *DC&R*. Nov–Dec 1982;25(8):772–777.

6. Ragnarsson-Olding BK, Nilsson PJ, Olding LB, Nilsson BR. Primary ano-rectal malignant melanomas within a population-based national patient series in Sweden during 40 years. *Acta Oncol (Stock)*. 2009;48(1):125–131.

7. Falch C, Stojadinovic A, Hann-von-Weyhern C, et al. Anorectal malignant melanoma: extensive 45-year review and proposal for a novel staging classification. *J Am Coll Surg*. Aug 2013;217(2):324–335.

8. Piura B. Management of primary melanoma of the female urogenital tract. *Lancet Oncol*. Oct 2008;9(10):973–981.

9. Curtin JA, Fridlyand J, Kageshita T, et al. Distinct sets of genetic alterations in melanoma. *N Engl J Med*. Nov 17, 2005;353(20):2135–2147.

10. Sekine S, Nakanishi Y, Ogawa R, Kouda S, Kanai Y. Esophageal melanomas harbor frequent *NRAS* mutations unlike melanomas of other mucosal sites. *Virchows Archiv*. May 1, 2009;454(5):513–517.

11. Omholt K, Grafstrom E, Kanter-Lewensohn L, Hansson J, Ragnarsson-Olding BK. *KIT* pathway alterations in mucosal melanomas of the vulva and other sites. *Clin Cancer Res*. Jun 15, 2011;17(12):3933–3942.

12. Curtin JA, Busam K, Pinkel D, Bastian BC. Somatic activation of *KIT* in distinct subtypes of melanoma. *J Clin Oncol*. Sep 10, 2006;24(26):4340–4346.

13. Antonescu CR, Busam KJ, Francone TD, et al. L576P *KIT* mutation in anal melanomas correlates with KIT protein expression and is sensitive to specific kinase inhibition. *Int J Cancer*. Jul 15, 2007;121(2):257–264.

14. Beadling C, Jacobson-Dunlop E, Hodi FS, et al. *KIT* gene mutations and copy number in melanoma subtypes. *Clin Cancer Res*. Nov 1, 2008;14(21):6821–6828.

15. Rivera RS, Nagatsuka H, Gunduz M, et al. C-kit protein expression correlated with activating mutations in *KIT* gene in oral mucosal melanoma. *Virchows Archiv*. Jan 2008;452(1):27–32.

16. Satzger I, Schaefer T, Kuettler U, et al. Analysis of c-KIT expression and *KIT* gene mutation in human mucosal melanomas. *Br J Cancer*. Dec 16, 2008;99(12):2065–2069.

17. Ballantyne AJ. Malignant melanoma of the skin of the head and neck. An analysis of 405 cases. *Am J Surg*. Oct 1970;120(4):425–431.

18. Prasad ML, Busam KJ, Patel SG, Hoshaw-Woodard S, Shah JP, Huvos AG. Clinicopathologic differences in malignant melanoma arising in oral squamous and sinonasal respiratory mucosa of the upper aerodigestive tract. *Arch Pathol Lab Med*. Aug 2003;127(8):997–1002.

19. Edge SBB, Byrd DR, Compton CC, Fritz AG, Greene FL, Trotti A, eds. *AJCC Cancer Staging Manual, 7th Edition*. 2010. Chicago IL: Springer and AJCC.

20. Moxley KM, Fader AN, Rose PG, et al. Malignant melanoma of the vulva: an extension of cutaneous melanoma? *Gynecol Oncol*. Sep 2011;122(3):612–617.

21. Mert I, Semaan A, Winer I, Morris RT, Ali-Fehmi R. Vulvar/vaginal melanoma: an updated surveillance epidemiology and end results database review, comparison with cutaneous melanoma and significance of racial disparities. *Int J Gynecol Cancer*. Jul 2013;23(6):1118–1125.

22. Thompson LD, Wieneke JA, Miettinen M. Sinonasal tract and nasopharyngeal melanomas: a clinicopathologic study of 115 cases with a proposed staging system. *Am J Surg Pathol*. May 2003;27(5):594–611.

23. Patel SG, Prasad ML, Escrig M, et al. Primary mucosal malignant melanoma of the head and neck. *Head & Neck*. Mar 2002;24(3):247–257.

24. Podnos YD, Tsai NC, Smith D, Ellenhorn JD. Factors affecting survival in patients with anal melanoma. *Am Surg*. Oct 2006;72(10):917–920.

25. Carvajal RD, Spencer SA, Lydiatt W. Mucosal melanoma: a clinically and biologically unique disease entity. *JNCCN*. Mar 2012;10(3):345–356.

28. Wushou A, Hou J, Zhao YJ, Miao XC. Postoperative adjuvant radiotherapy improves loco-regional recurrence of head and neck mucosal melanoma. *Journal of cranio-maxillo-facial surgery : official publication of the European Association for Cranio-Maxillo-Facial Surgery*. May 2015;43(4):553–558.

27. Yeh JJ, Shia J, Hwu WJ, et al. The role of abdominoperineal resection as surgical therapy for anorectal melanoma. *Ann Surg*. Dec 2006;244(6):1012–1017.

28. Sugiyama VE, Chan JK, Shin JY, Berek JS, Osann K, Kapp DS. Vulvar melanoma: a multivariable analysis of 644 patients. *Obstet Gynecol*. Aug 2007;110(2 Pt 1):296–301.

29. Moreno MA, Hanna EY. Management of mucosal melanomas of the head and neck: did we make any progress? *Curr Opin Otolaryngol Head Neck Surg*. Apr 2010;18(2):101–106.

30. Owens JM, Roberts DB, Myers JN. The role of postoperative adjuvant radiation therapy in the treatment of mucosal melanomas of the head and neck region. *Arch Otolaryngol Head Neck Surg*. Aug 2003;129(8):864–868.

31. Temam S, Mamelle G, Marandas P, et al. Postoperative radiotherapy for primary mucosal melanoma of the head and neck. *Cancer*. Jan 15, 2005;103(2):313–319.

32. Kelly P, Zagars GK, Cormier JN, Ross MI, Guadagnolo BA. Sphincter-sparing local excision and hypofractionated radiation therapy for anorectal melanoma: a 20-year experience. *Cancer*. Oct 15, 2011;117(20):4747–4755.

33. Ballo MT, Gershenwald JE, Zagars GK, et al. Sphincter-sparing local excision and adjuvant radiation for anal-rectal melanoma. *J Clin Oncol*. Dec 1, 2002;20(23):4555–4558.

34. Lian B, Si L, Cui C, et al. Phase II randomized trial comparing high-dose IFN-α2b with temozolomide plus cisplatin as systemic adjuvant therapy for resected mucosal melanoma. *Clin Cancer Res*. Aug 15, 2013;19(16):4488–4498.

35. Hodi FS, O'Day SJ, McDermott DF, et al. Improved survival with ipilimumab in patients with metastatic melanoma. *N Engl J Med*. Aug 19, 2010;363(8):711–723.

36. Wolchok JD, Kluger H, Callahan MK, et al. Nivolumab plus ipilimumab in advanced melanoma. *N Engl J Med*. Jul 11, 2013;369(2):122–133.

37. Del Vecchio M, Di Guardo L, Ascierto PA, et al. Efficacy and safety of ipilimumab 3mg/kg in patients with pretreated, metastatic, mucosal melanoma. *Eur J Cancer*. Jan 2014;50(1):121–127.

38. Postow MA, Luke JJ, Bluth MJ, et al. Ipilimumab for patients with advanced mucosal melanoma. *Oncologist*. Jun 2013;18(6):726–732.

39. Carvajal RD, Antonescu CR, Wolchok JD, al. E. KIT as a therapeutic target in metastatic melanoma. *JAMA*. Jun 8, 2011;305(22):2327–2334.

40. Guo J, Si L, Kong Y, et al. Phase II, open-label, single-arm trial of imatinib mesylate in patients with metastatic melanoma harboring c-Kit mutation or amplification. *J Clin Oncol*. Jul 20, 2011;29(21):2904–2909.

41. Hodi FS, Corless CL, Giobbie-Hurder A, et al. Imatinib for melanomas harboring mutationally activated or amplified KIT arising on mucosal, acral, and chronically sun-damaged skin. *J Clin Oncol*. Sep 10, 2013;31(26):3182–3190.

42. Singh AD, Turell ME, Topham AK. Uveal melanoma: trends in incidence, treatment, and survival. *Ophthalmology*. Sep 2011;118(9):1881–1885.

43. Rietschel P, Panageas KS, Hanlon C, Patel A, Abramson DH, Chapman PB. Variates of survival in metastatic uveal melanoma. *J Clin Oncol*. Nov 1, 2005;23(31):8076–8080.

44. The Collaborative Ocular Melanoma Study Group. Assessment of metastatic disease status at death in 435 patients with large choroidal melanoma in the Collaborative Ocular Melanoma Study (COMS): COMS Report no. 15. *Arch Ophthalmol*. 2001;119(5):670–676.

45. Rietschel P, Panageas KS, Hanlon C, Patel A, Abramson DH, Chapman PB. Variates of survival in metastatic uveal melanoma. *J Clin Oncol*. 2005;23(31):8076–8080.

46. Bedikian AY, Papadopoulos N, Plager C, Eton O, Ring S. Phase II evaluation of temozolomide in metastatic choroidal melanoma. *Melanoma Res*. Jun 2003;13(3):303–306.

47. Kujala E, Damato B, Coupland SE, et al. Staging of ciliary body and choroidal melanomas based on anatomic extent. *J Clin Oncol*. Aug 1, 2013;31(22):2825–2831.

48. Shields CL, Kaliki S, Furuta M, Fulco E, Alarcon C, Shields JA. American Joint Committee on Cancer Classification of posterior uveal melanoma (tumor size category) predicts prognosis in 7731 patients. *Ophthalmology*. Oct 2013;120(10):2066–2071.

49. Bornfeld N, Prescher G, Becher R, Hirche H, Jöckel KH, Horsthemke B. Prognostic implications of monosomy 3 in uveal melanoma. *Lancet*. 1996;347(9010):1222–1225.

50. Sisley K, Rennie IG, Parsons MA, et al. Abnormalities of chromosomes 3 and 8 in posterior uveal melanoma correlate with prognosis. *Genes Chromosomes Cancer*. May 1997;19(1):22–28.

51. Onken MD, Worley LA, Char DH, et al. Collaborative Ocular Oncology Group Report number 1: Prospective validation of a multi-gene prognostic assay in uveal melanoma. *Ophthalmology*. 8//2012;119(8):1596–1603.

52. Francis JH, Patel SP, Gombos DS, Carvajal RD. Surveillance options for patients with uveal melanoma following definitive management. *American Society of Clinical Oncology educational book/ASCO. American Society of Clinical Oncology. Meeting*. 2013:382–287.

53. Strobel K, Bode B, Dummer R, et al. Limited value of 18F-FDG PET/CT and S-100B tumour marker in the detection of liver metastases from uveal melanoma compared to liver metastases from cutaneous melanoma. *Eur J Nucl Med Mol Imaging*. Nov 2009;36(11):1774–1782.

54. Adams KS, Abramson DH, Ellsworth RM, et al. Cobalt plaque versus enucleation for uveal melanoma: comparison of survival rates. *Br J Ophthalmol*. Jul 1988;72(7):494–497.

55. Augsburger JJ, Correa ZM, Freire J, Brady LW. Long-term survival in choroidal and ciliary body melanoma after enucleation versus plaque radiation therapy. *Ophthalmology*. Sep 1998;105(9):1670–1678.

56. Seddon JM, Gragoudas ES, Egan KM, et al. Relative survival rates after alternative therapies for uveal melanoma. *Ophthalmology*. Jun 1990;97(6):769–777.

57. Collaborative Ocular Melanoma Study (COMS). The COMS randomized trial of iodine 125 brachytherapy for choroidal melanoma: V. Twelve-year mortality rates and prognostic factors: COMS Report no. 28. *Arch Ophthalmol*. Dec 2006;124(12):1684–1693.

58. Diener-West M, Earle JD, Fine SL, et al. The COMS randomized trial of iodine 125 brachytherapy for choroidal melanoma, III: initial mortality findings. COMS Report no. 18. *Arch Ophthalmol*. Jul 2001;119(7):969–982.

59. Hawkins BS. The Collaborative Ocular Melanoma Study (COMS) randomized trial of pre-enucleation radiation of large choroidal melanoma: IV. Ten-year mortality findings and prognostic factors. COMS Report no. 24. *Am J Ophthalmol*. Dec 2004;138(6):936–951.

60. Collaborative Ocular Melanoma Study. Development of metastatic disease after enrollment in the coms trials for treatment of choroidal melanoma: Collaborative Ocular Melanoma Study Group Report no. 26. *Arch Ophthalmol*. 2005;123(12):1639–1643.

61. Salmon RJ, Levy C, Plancher C, et al. Treatment of liver metastases from uveal melanoma by combined surgery-chemotherapy. *Eur J Surg Oncol*. Apr 1998;24(2):127–130.

62. Ackerman NB, Lien WM, Silverman NA. The blood supply of experimental liver metastases. 3. The effects of acute ligation of the hepatic artery or portal vein. *Surgery*. Apr 1972;71(4):636–641.

63. Breedis C, Young G. The blood supply of neoplasms in the liver. *Am J Pathol*. Sep-Oct 1954;30(5):969–977.

64. Lien WM, Ackerman NB. The blood supply of experimental liver metastases. II. A microcirculatory study of the normal and tumor vessels of the liver with the use of perfused silicone rubber. *Surgery*. Aug 1970;68(2):334–340.

65. Sato T. Locoregional management of hepatic metastasis from primary uveal melanoma. *Semin Oncol*. Apr 2010;37(2):127–138.

66. Pingpank JF, Hughes MS, Alexander HR, et al. A phase III random assignment trial comparing percutaneous hepatic perfusion with melphalan (PHP-mel) to standard of care for patients with hepatic metastases from metastatic ocular or cutaneous melanoma. *J Clin Oncol*. 2010;28(18 suppl):LBA8512. Abstract.

67. Leyvraz S, Suciu S, Piperno-Neumann S, et al. Randomized phase III trial of intravenous (IV) versus hepatic intra-arterial (HIA) fotemustine in patients with liver metastases from uveal melanoma: Final results of the EORTC 18021 study. *J Clin Oncol*. 2012;30(Suppl; abstract 8532).

68. Bedikian AY, Legha SS, Mavligit G, et al. Treatment of uveal melanoma metastatic to the liver: a review of the M. D. Anderson Cancer Center experience and prognostic factors. *Cancer*. Nov 1, 1995;76(9):1665–1670.

69. Homsi J, Bedikian AY, Papadopoulos NE, et al. Phase 2 open-label study of weekly docosahexaenoic acid-paclitaxel in patients with metastatic uveal melanoma. *Melanoma Res*. Dec 2010;20(6):507–510.

70. Kivela T, Suciu S, Hansson J, et al. Bleomycin, vincristine, lomustine and dacarbazine (BOLD) in combination with recombinant interferon alpha-2b for metastatic uveal melanoma. *Eur J Cancer*. May 2003;39(8):1115–1120.

71. O'Neill PA, Butt M, Eswar CV, Gillis P, Marshall E. A prospective single arm phase II study of dacarbazine and treosulfan as first-line therapy in metastatic uveal melanoma. *Melanoma Res*. Jun 2006;16(3):245–248.

72. Penel N, Delcambre C, Durando X, et al. O-Mel-Inib: a Cancero-pole Nord-Ouest multicenter phase II trial of high-dose imatinib mesylate in metastatic uveal melanoma. *Invest New Drugs*. Dec 2008;26(6):561–565.

73. Schmidt-Hieber M, Schmittel A, Thiel E, Keilholz U. A phase II study of bendamustine chemotherapy as second-line treatment in metastatic uveal melanoma. *Melanoma Res*. Dec 2004;14(6):439–442.

74. Schmittel A, Scheulen ME, Bechrakis NE, et al. Phase II trial of cisplatin, gemcitabine and treosulfan in patients with metastatic uveal melanoma. *Melanoma Res.* Jun 2005;15(3):205–207.

75. Schmittel A, Schmidt-Hieber M, Martus P, et al. A randomized phase II trial of gemcitabine plus treosulfan versus treosulfan alone in patients with metastatic uveal melanoma. *Ann Oncol.* Dec 2006;17(12):1826–1829.

76. Mahipal A, Tijani L, Chan K, Laudadio M, Mastrangelo MJ, Sato T. A pilot study of sunitinib malate in patients with metastatic uveal melanoma. *Melanoma Res.* Dec 2012;22(6):440–446.

77. Sacco JJ, Nathan PD, Danson S, et al.. Sunitinib versus dacarbazine as first-line treatment in patients with metastatic uveal melanoma. *J Clin Oncol.* 2013;31(Suppl; Abstract 9031).

78. Kelderman S, van der Kooij MK, van den Eertwegh AJ, et al. Ipilimumab in pretreated metastatic uveal melanoma patients. Results of the Dutch Working Group on Immunotherapy of Oncology (WIN-O). *Acta Oncol (Stock).* Nov 2013;52(8):1786–1788.

79. Khattak MA, Fisher R, Hughes P, Gore M, Larkin J. Ipilimumab activity in advanced uveal melanoma. *Melanoma Res.* Feb 2013;23(1):79–81.

80. Luke JJ, Callahan MK, Postow MA, et al. Clinical activity of ipilimumab for metastatic uveal melanoma: A retrospective review of the Dana-Farber Cancer Institute, Massachusetts General Hospital, Memorial Sloan-Kettering Cancer Center, and University Hospital of Lausanne experience. *Cancer.* Oct 15, 2013;119(20):3687–3695.

81. Maio M, Danielli R, Chiarion-Sileni V, et al. Efficacy and safety of ipilimumab in patients with pre-treated, uveal melanoma. *Ann Oncol.* Nov 2013;24(11):2911–2915.

82. Van Raamsdonk CD, Bezrookove V, Green G, et al. Frequent somatic mutations of *GNAQ* in uveal melanoma and blue naevi. *Nature.* Jan 29, 2009;457(7229):599–602.

83. Van Raamsdonk CD, Griewank KG, Crosby MB, et al. Mutations in *GNA11* in uveal melanoma. *N Engl J Med.* Dec 2, 2010;363(23):2191–2199.

84. Patel M, Smyth E, Chapman PB, et al. Therapeutic implications of the emerging molecular biology of uveal melanoma. *Clin Cancer Res.* Apr 15, 2011;17(8):2087–2100.

85. Carvajal RD, Sosman JA, Quevedo JF, et al. Effect of selumetinib vs chemotherapy on progression-free survival in uveal melanoma: a randomized clinical trial. *JAMA.* Jun 18, 2014;311(23):2397–2405.

86. Snyder A, Makarov V, Merghoub T, et al. Genetic basis for clinical response to CTLA-4 blockade in melanoma. *N Engl J Med.* Dec 4, 2014;371(23):2189–2199.

87. Furney SJ, Pedersen M, Gentien D, et al. *SF3B1* mutations are associated with alternative splicing in uveal melanoma. *Cancer Discov.* Oct 2013;3(10):1122–1129.

Chapter 13

Special Considerations in the Management of Pediatric Melanoma Patients

Damon Reed and Fariba Navid

The diagnosis and workup of melanoma in a child is often a complex process. The pathological studies, staging, surgical management, and decisions about adjuvant therapy are often based on extrapolation from adult data. At the same time, the risks and benefits of these decisions are magnified by the patient's young age and long life expectancy.

Melanoma is the most common primary malignant tumor of the skin in children, accounting for 1.4% of new cancer diagnoses in patients less than 20 years of age.[1] In subgroup analysis, melanoma contributes to less than 1% of all malignant diagnoses in children less than 15 years of age, but to 7% of all malignant diagnoses in 15- to 19-year-olds.[2] In the USA while the incidence of other pediatric malignancies has remained stable, the incidence of adolescent melanoma is increasing at a rate of 2% per year without a corresponding increase in mortality.[1,3]

Clinical Presentation

The index of suspicion may be the most important contributor to detection of possible melanoma during the physical examination. Perhaps because pediatric melanoma is perceived to be rare and unexpected, the average time to diagnosis is reported to be as long as nine months.[4] Interestingly, a much higher number of nevi are resected per melanoma diagnosis in pediatrics (nearly 600, 20 times the number in adults), perhaps because the consequences of overlooking a malignancy are amplified in very young patients.[5] In patients under 10 years of age, as many as a third of melanomas arise from large congenital nevi. These cases carry the risk of central nervous system involvement, which is very difficult to treat.[6]

While the traditional ABCDEs of the melanoma exam remain important in pediatrics, there can be substantially more variation in the presentation and diagnosis. In reporting a large cohort study, the authors recommended that additional ABCD criteria, namely Amelanotic, Bump/Bleeding, Color uniformity, and De novo/any Diameter be considered for children.[7] This proposal was based on a review of 70 pediatric patients with melanoma (19 who

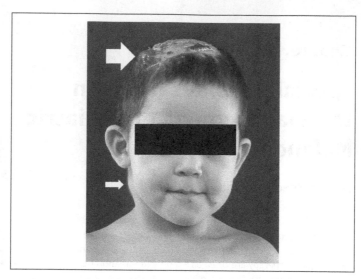

Figure 13.1 Four-year-old Hispanic male with a 6-month history of soft, non-tender, pruritic nodules (thick arrow) arising from a giant congenital nevus of the scalp and a 3-month history of palpable right cervical lymphadenopathy (thin arrow). A partial resection of the nodular masses of the scalp was performed. The pathology was consistent with malignant melanoma.

were age 10 years or younger) in which the majority of both age groups, <10 and >10 years, had raised lesions (*B*ump), uniform or no *C*olor, *D*iameter < 6 mm, *D*e novo lesion, and *E*volution. Most patients <10 years of age had Amelanotic lesions.[7] A case-matched study of melanoma in pediatric patients and matched adults showed a higher incidence of family history of melanoma and atypical nevi or dysplastic nevus syndrome in the pediatric group, suggesting that melanoma in the young has a genetic component.[8] Eleven of the 73 pediatric patients had development of a melanoma within a congenital nevus (Figure 13.1), as compared to only 2 of the 146 adults; furthermore, more children than adults had a precursor lesion.[8] However, another study found that common nevi are not significantly more frequent in pediatric patients with melanoma.[9]

Predisposing Factors

Most pediatric melanomas are sporadic, although certain predisposing factors unique to children should be considered. These include congenital melanoma syndromes that consist of giant congenital nevi and DNA-repair defects. Congenital melanocytic nevi (CMN) are benign melanocyte proliferations that present at birth or shortly thereafter and are categorized on the basis of size. The reported incidence of malignant transformation of CMN is diverse; small (<1.5 cm in diameter) and medium (1.5–20 cm)-sized CMN have a reported lifetime risk of malignant transformation of 2–5%, typically after adolescence.[10,11] In contrast, giant CMN (>20 cm in diameter) carry a reported risk ranging from 5–40%, which is greatest in the first decade of life.[10,12] Approximately one third of prepubertal melanomas arise from large congenital nevi.[13] In a collection of retrospective reviews that reported the association of melanoma with congenital nevi, 45 out of 693 (6.4%) patients had a congenital nevus that preceded the diagnosis.[14] Melanoma arising from a CMN seems to have distinct pathophysiology with absence of TERT promoter mutations and presence of NRAS activating mutations in a small series(Lu et al).[14a]

Sensitivity to DNA damage, mutations in cell cycle tumor suppressor genes, and mutations in other tumor suppressor genes are associated with a greater risk of melanoma. However, most pediatric melanomas are not explained by known genetic disorders, either individually or collectively.[15] Xeroderma pigmentosum is a disorder of nucleotide excision repair. Because of their sensitivity to DNA damage caused by ultraviolet radiation, affected patients have a 5–13% risk of developing melanoma before their 20th birthday.[16, 17] The mutational landscape of a cohort of pediatric melanoma has more recently been explored with clear differences between conventional melanoma and melanomas arising from congenital nevi or spitzoid melanomas.[14a] While pediatric melanoma shared genetic changes with adult melanoma with BRAF V600 mutations in a majority of cases and >80% of single-nucleotide variants being consistent with UV damage, an addition finding was of TERT promoter mutations in all 15 cases. TERT promoter mutation was only seen in 1 of 5 spitzoid melanomas, the only one to metastasize. Mutations in the cell cycle genes CDKN2A or CDK4 can also lead to multiple and recurrent melanomas, but they are present in less than 5% of childhood melanomas.[16] Dysplastic nevi also suggest the risk of melanoma and of a familial melanoma syndrome. Familial melanoma remains incompletely understood, but it accounts for 5–10% of cases of pediatric melanoma.

Evaluation and Staging

A biopsy of all suspicious lesions should be obtained and evaluated by a dermatopathologist with expertise in pediatric dermatopathology. However, even with this strategy, challenges are likely to arise after the biopsy. While a pathologist can clearly differentiate a normal nevus from melanoma, the spectrum of histological, immunohistochemical, and genetic differences between normal and malignant lesions seems to be especially broad in pediatric cases. Many pediatric lesions are unequivocally malignant melanoma, while others, collectively termed "atypical melanocytic proliferations" (AMPs), are more ambiguous and have been the subject of much debate.[18, 19] They carry names such as "Spitzoid tumor of uncertain malignant potential," "melanocytic tumor of uncertain malignant potential," "superficial atypical melanocytic proliferation of uncertain significance," and "atypical Spitzoid tumor."[19] Expert, comprehensive pathological review is needed to minimize the likelihood of under-treatment of atypical lesions that will ultimately be recategorized as melanoma, often too late. Table 13.1 lists various immunohistochemical

Table 13.1 Pathological Techniques for Differentiating Melanoma from Atypical Melanocytic Proliferations in Children

Method	Marker	Protein Type	Comments
IHC	HMB-45	Melanocytic marker	Protein related to melanosomes that typically diminishes in staining intensity as a melanocytic proliferation "matures."
			Useful in identifying Spitzoid lesions, in which expression is lower or absent at the base of the lesions, whereas typical melanomas show diffuse expression throughout the dermal component.
IHC	p16	Cell cycle protein	Commonly absent in malignant melanoma but present in many Spitz nevi and compound nevi.[18]
IHC	Ki-67	Measure of cellular proliferation	Ki-67 expression increases progressively from Spitz nevi (5.04%) to atypical Spitz nevi (10%) to cutaneous melanoma (36.88%).[19]
IHC	Phospho-histone H3	Measure of cellular proliferation	Specific for cells in active mitosis. Significantly lower mitotic index in Spitz nevi than in melanoma.
CGH	–	–	Available only in the research setting, and significantly more time-consuming and technically difficult.[20] 11q gain is suggestive of Spitz nevi rather than melanoma.[21]
FISH	–	–	Offers the advantage of four color-specific probes and can be performed on FFPE tissue. While the original report showed a sensitivity of 80%, subsequent independent analyses with longer follow-up have demonstrated somewhat lower sensitivity and specificity.
IHC of Lymph Nodes	p16 and Ki-67	–	Advocated for evaluation of equivocal nodes; the absence of p16 staining and/or elevated Ki-67 staining favor a diagnosis of metastatic melanoma.
Sequencing	HRAS	Oncoprotein	HRAS mutations are exclusive to Spitz nevi and are not seen in pediatric melanoma.[22,23]

Abbreviations: HMB-45, Human Melanoma Black-45; IHC, immunohistochemistry; CGH, comparative genomic hybridization; FFPE, fresh-frozen, paraffin-embedded.

and molecular markers that have been reported as helpful in categorizing an atypical lesion. There is no reliable method to assess the natural history of diagnostically challenging lesions, as metastatic spread reclassifies an atypical lesion as a melanoma. In at least one series, patients with AMPs that were later reclassified as melanomas actually had lower survival estimates than did patients initially diagnosed with melanoma.[20] The phenomenon of AMPs is limited to pediatric and young adult patients and does not typically occur after the third decade of life.

Teamwork, emphasizing communication, proper biopsy technique, and correct specimen processing constitute the optimal approach to pathological evaluation of a clinically suspect pigmented lesion in a child. The most desirable biopsy method is excision. However, many lesions are biopsied using the shave or punch biopsy techniques. Formalin fixation is sufficient for all routine and specialized specimen evaluation methods, including fluorescence *in situ* hybridization (FISH) and comparative genomic hybridization. Specimens should be submitted to a laboratory that employs a board-certified dermatopathologist, preferably one with expertise in the pediatric age group. To assure good communication with the pathologist, the requisition should state the patient's age; the site, color, and size of the lesion; and whether the biopsy specimen comprises the entire lesion. A history of congenital nevus in the area biopsied should be noted, as well as any recent changes or antecedent trauma. Ideally, a photograph of the lesion *in situ* should be submitted with the biopsy.

The pathology report should include a microscopic description, final diagnosis, and microstaging data, as recommended for adult melanoma. Microstaging data include histological subtype, Clark's level (invasion depth), Breslow level (lesion thickness), mitoses/mm^2, growth phase (radial or vertical), and the presence or absence of ulceration, regression, angiolymphatic invasion, perineural invasion, and/or a benign precursor lesion. It should be noted whether the lesion extends past the biopsy margin. The value of a second and, if necessary, third opinion in cases of suspected pediatric melanoma cannot be overemphasized. Although the pathological diagnosis of such cases can be difficult and the subject of great discussion, the majority of pediatric melanomas do not differ histopathologically from adult melanomas. Approximately 60% are of the superficial, spreading subtype, while the nodular subtype is more abundant in children than in adults.[14, 21] Spitzoid melanoma is also more abundant in children and has a higher rate of positive sentinel lymph nodes. While the optimal management of atypical melanocytic proliferations is controversial, clear cases of melanoma are staged and managed similarly to their adult counterparts. Decisions regarding sentinel lymph node biopsy are relatively straightforward in adults and depend mainly on the thickness of the melanoma. Ideally, the sentinel lymph node is biopsied at the time of primary tumor resection. In practice, however, the diagnosis of melanoma is unexpected, and thus a re-resection with wide margins is usually paired with the sentinel lymph node biopsy. It is well established that the rate of sentinel node involvement is higher in pediatric melanoma (approximately 25–40%) than in adult melanoma which is 12–16%.[22–24] Sentinel lymph node biopsy is well-tolerated, and in the appropriate context, it can provide a wealth of information. A negative sentinel node provides reassurance. Even though the frequency of positive sentinel nodes is higher than in adults, most pediatric patients are node-negative and have an excellent prognosis.[25]

A positive sentinel lymph node biopsy, on the other hand, provides important prognostic information and prompts the creation of a defined therapeutic plan. In a single institution's experience with unequivocal pediatric melanoma, the majority of patients who experienced recurrence had node-positive disease.[26] The diagnosis of metastatic melanoma in lymph nodes can be challenging. Benign nevus cells, including cells from Spitz nevi or cellular blue nevi, can normally be found in lymph nodes draining the skin. Hence, the presence of nevus cells in a node is not proof of a metastatic lesion. The criteria that distinguish between nodal melanoma involvement and benign nodal nevi or nests remain the subject of debate. Multiple positive nodes, expansile nodal lesions, and/or lesions with parenchymal deposits or necrosis are highly suggestive of melanoma.

While minimal morbidity follows sentinel lymph node biopsy, completion lymphadenectomy can cause substantially more morbidity, depending on its location. A positive sentinel node raises the suspicion of nodal disease in the remainder of the basin. The decision to perform a completion lymphadenectomy involves careful weighing of the risks and benefits and is often discussed by a team of experienced physicians. The morbidity associated with completion lymphadenectomy, especially in the inguinal and axillary regions, must be balanced with the anticipated benefits of the procedure. In most cases, the arguments for and against completion lymphadenectomy are similar to those in adults.[27, 28]

Ultrasound, CT, MRI, and PET imaging are appropriate for use in staging and should be considered in view of the anatomical coverage needed. Lymph node basins should be carefully assessed in all cases; when basins are equivocal or suspect, ultrasound-guided needle aspiration or removal of the questionable lymph node(s) should be considered for pathological evaluation. Despite the risks associated with ionizing radiation, we routinely use diagnostic imaging, such as PET/CT scans, in the work-up of melanomas with high-risk features such as CLARK level IV-V or clinical concern for metastasis.[29]

Prognosis

In children and adolescents, as in adults, the outcome of melanoma is stage-dependent.[30–32] Data from the Surveillance, Epidemiology, and End Results (SEER) database showed 5-year melanoma-specific survival to be 96.1%±1.5% for localized disease, 77.2%±9.3% for regional disease, and 57.3%±21.3% for distant disease in 1,255 patients under 20 years of age.[31] In the U.S. National Cancer Database, the 5-year overall survival estimate was 93.6%±0.9% for localized disease, 68.0%±4.2% for regional disease, but 11.8%±6.4% for distant disease in 3,158 patients ages 1 to 19 years with cutaneous melanoma.[30] In both of these registry-based analyses, the outcome of patients more than 10 years of age was similar to that in patients 20 to 24 years of age. However, in the U.S. National Cancer Database analysis, outcome was worse in patients under 10 years of age than in the older age groups. In contrast, SEER data showed an outcome similar to that of the older age groups despite poor prognostic features (thicker lesions, more frequent distant disease, and nodular histology). The finding of a comparable or better outcome in younger, prepubertal children than in older children and adults, despite high-risk features, has been noted in smaller series[32–35] and suggests that the biological behavior of these tumors differs from that of adult-type melanoma. Furthermore, the American Joint Committee on Cancer (AJCC) staging system, which relies heavily on clinicopathological criteria, was validated in adults but may not be applicable to children. Especially in the case of lesions that are not clearly melanoma whereby single lymph node positivity does not confer the same prognostic significance.

Treatment

Surgery is the mainstay of treatment for localized cutaneous melanoma. Surgical management in children integrates lymphoscintigraphy with sentinel node biopsy for staging, prognostication, and selection of additional therapy. Most centers perform sentinel node biopsy on the basis of lesion thickness (>0.75–1 mm) or the presence of histological features suggestive of a more aggressive tumor (e.g., ulceration, increased mitotic rate, angiolymphatic invasion). Close observation alone is indicated in patients with no evidence of tumor in the sentinel node and absence of distant metastases. If the sentinel lymph node does harbor tumor cells, complete lymph node dissection is recommended, and the risks and benefits of adjuvant interferon therapy are discussed with the family.

Three studies have been reported to date evaluating the feasibility in children with resected stage III melanoma of using the high-dose interferon "Kirkwood" regimen.[36] Chao et al.[4] conducted a retrospective review of 12 patients treated at the University of Michigan over a 14-year period. These patients tolerated the therapy well and required fewer dose modifications than reported in adult studies. The second study was another retrospective review of 11 patients with melanoma who underwent sentinel lymph node biopsy at the Hospital for Sick Children in Toronto[37]; five patients consented to interferon therapy based on the Kirkwood regimen. Dose modification was required by two patients during induction therapy and by two patients during maintenance therapy (for abnormal liver function indicators); depression and major mood change were observed in two patients. The third study, at St. Jude Children's Research Hospital (Memphis, Tennessee, U.S.A.),[38] prospectively assessed the Kirkwood regimen in 15 newly diagnosed patients ≤18 years of age with resected regional lymph node disease. While the frequencies of toxicities were different between adults and children, new adverse events were not seen in children. Whereas constitutional symptoms are the most commonly reported grade 3/4 toxicities in adults, neutropenia was the most common grade 3/4 toxicity in children, followed by elevated hepatic transaminases. All toxicities were reversible and required interruption of therapy or dose modification. No patients were taken off study because of interferon-related toxicity. Like Chao et al.,[4] the authors reported fewer dose modifications than in adult trials, during both induction and maintenance therapy. Because of the small number of patients in these studies, the benefit of interferon therapy in children remains unknown.

Although interferon α-2b is well tolerated in children, subcutaneous injection of the medication three times weekly is inconvenient. A newer formulation, incorporating a polyethylene glycol (PEG) molecule bound to interferon alpha(symbol)-2b, demonstrates better tolerability and perhaps better efficacy[39–46].

A current pediatric clinical trial (NCT00539591) is comparing the pharmacokinetics, feasibility, and quality-of-life impact of subcutaneous peginterferon 1 mcg/kg/week for 48 weeks with that of conventional interferon during maintenance therapy. Results favoring the use of peginterferon once weekly would certainly increase the convenience of therapy, especially in children.

Metastatic or recurrent melanoma carries a dismal prognosis. Promising therapies being developed in adults but not currently on label for pediatric patients include checkpoint inhibitors and agents targeting the most common mutation in melanoma, BRAF V600E.[46a–q] Patients should be encouraged to participate in a clinical trial, if one is available. However, few novel therapies are available for these patients. With the increasing incidence of melanoma in adolescents and the growing array of treatment options, there is a conceptual shift toward the evaluation of new agents during earlier phases of drug development in this patient group. Suggested strategies have included lowering the age of eligibility and opening stand-alone trials for this age group. Two pharmaceutical company–sponsored, multi-institutional, international trials are under way for patients 12–18 years of age with metastatic or recurrent melanoma: a phase I/II study of vemurafenib for patients with *BRAF*-mutated melanoma (NCT01519323) and a phase II study of ipilimumab (NCT01696045). Options for younger patients, those who do not qualify, or those unable to access these trials include off-label use of these commercially available drugs, high-dose interleukin-2, dacarbazine, temozolomide, or biochemotherapy.

Follow-up

No guidelines have been established for follow-up of children diagnosed with melanoma. Because surgical resection remains the most effective treatment, early detection of recurrence or of a new primary melanoma may improve prognosis. For this reason, an important aspect of follow-up is education of parents and patients about regular self-examination of skin and lymph nodes, and regular follow-up clinic visits that include a comprehensive history and physical examination. The interval between visits is usually influenced by the risk of recurrence, family history of melanoma, presence of atypical or dysplastic moles, and family/patient reliability and concerns. Our practice is to initially evaluate patients at three-month intervals. Patients should be followed for more than five years, since late recurrence has been reported.[21]

The role of routine laboratory and imaging studies in adults is controversial. The argument against performing these studies routinely is that they have a low yield and a relatively high false-positive rate. The most recent National Comprehensive Cancer Network (NCCN) guidelines recommend that these studies be considered only in patients at high risk (AJCC Stage IIB to IV) or who have signs and/or symptoms. The recommended imaging during the first five years of follow-up is PET/CT or CT scans every 3 to 12 months and an annual brain MRI. Consideration could also be given to use ultrasound as a tool to monitor a lymph node basin with a negative sentinel lymph node or with a shallow depth.[47] These are reasonable guidelines for children at high risk of recurrence. However, it is important to balance the potential benefit of imaging with the negative effects of added radiation exposure or the need for sedation, especially in children. The only study specifically investigating the utility of routine diagnostic imaging during follow-up of children with malignant melanoma was a retrospective review of 33 children treated over three decades at a single institution. All of the patients had deep or unknown primary lesions, indicating high-risk disease.[48] Routine imaging identified clinically undetectable metastases in 25% of the patients.

Further study is warranted in children. As new agents are approved and options for patients with metastatic melanoma go beyond surgical resection, the follow-up recommendations for adults and children should be reassessed. It is increasingly evident that the targeted immune approaches, such as anti-CTLA4 and anti-PD1 antibodies, may be most effective when the disease burden is low.

Future Directions

Although some progress has been made in understanding the epidemiology and biology of malignant melanoma in children, studies are limited by small patient numbers and by incomplete data in the large tumor registries. A more comprehensive understanding of the disease will require international collaboration committed to the collection and analysis of tumor samples and clinical data, including patient demographics and family history, and central review of pathology, treatment, and outcome. The same type of collaboration will be required to answer questions about the role of sentinel lymph node biopsy and complete lymph node dissection in children and to establish guidelines for staging at diagnosis and follow-up. Investment in this type of network could also support clinical trials that may reveal more appropriate strategies for the evaluation and treatment of pediatric melanoma.

With the recognition of a rising incidence of melanoma in the adolescent population, progress has been made in developing clinical trials for this age group, such as those described above. However, there remains an unmet need in this population as well as the younger age groups.[48a] What we are learning from the ongoing vemurafenib (NCT01519323) and ipilimumab (NCT01696045) trials for ages 12–18 years is that novel treatments must be made accessible to the entire pediatric and adolescent population early during drug development to meet accrual goals and maintain the interest of patients and families.

Finally, general pediatricians and pediatric oncologists can make their greatest contribution by using every opportunity to educate and remind patients about the importance of minimizing risk factors, including sun exposure and artificial tanning, and the benefits of early detection by regular skin self-examination. These measures are especially important in groups at high risk, such as children and adolescents with xeroderma pigmentosum, previous skin cancer, a family history of melanoma, giant congenital nevi, suspicious nevi, immunosuppression, genetic predisposition, or exposure to radiation.

Conclusion

While pediatric melanoma may be associated with familial syndromes or congenital nevi, it is most often sporadic, occurring after sun exposure in patients with a low skin phototype. The rarity of this disorder in pediatric patients demands astute clinical attention and a high index of suspicion for atypical lesions. The challenges range from the decision to biopsy to an often-equivocal pathological diagnosis. Several dedicated dermatopathologists are often consulted, and advanced techniques may be employed in selected circumstances. Deep lesions provide sufficient evidence to proceed to staging biopsy of sentinel lymph nodes. There is a clear trend toward a higher rate of positive sentinel lymph nodes in pediatric vs. adult patients with otherwise similar lesions. Conversely, outcomes in children, especially the very young (<10 years/prepubescent), are clearly superior to those of similarly staged adults. In view of the multiple variables involved and the limited quantity of good prospective data, clinical decisions in pediatric melanoma are challenging. Multidisciplinary care with excellent communication including a dermatopathologist with pediatric experience, surgeon, pediatric and medical oncologist is ideal in the management of pediatric melanoma.

References

1. Wong JR, Harris JK, Rodriguez-Galindo C, Johnson KJ. Incidence of childhood and adolescent melanoma in the United States: 1973–2009. *Pediatrics.* 2013;131(5):846–854.

2. Neier M, Pappo A, Navid F. Management of melanomas in children and young adults. *J Pediatr Hematol Oncol.* 2012;34(Suppl 2):S51–S54.

3. Lewis KG. Trends in pediatric melanoma mortality in the United States, 1968 through 2004. *Dermatol Surg.* 2008;34(2):152–159.

4. Chao MM, Schwartz JL, Wechsler DS, Thornburg CD, Griffith KA, Williams JA. High-risk surgically resected pediatric melanoma and adjuvant interferon therapy. *Pediatr Blood Cancer.* 2005;44(5):441–448.

5. Moscarella E, Zalaudek I, Cerroni L, et al. Excised melanocytic lesions in children and adolescents—a 10-year survey. *Br J Dermatol.* 2012;167(2):368–373.

6. Trozak DJ, Rowland WD, Hu F. Metastatic malignant melanoma in prepubertal children. *Pediatrics.* 1975;55(2):191–204.

7. Cordoro KM, Gupta D, Frieden IJ, McCalmont T, Kashani-Sabet M. Pediatric melanoma: results of a large cohort study and proposal for modified ABCD detection criteria for children. *J Am Acad Dermatol.* 2013;68(6):913–925.

8. Livestro DP, Kaine EM, Michaelson JS, et al. Melanoma in the young: differences and similarities with adult melanoma: a case-matched controlled analysis. *Cancer.* 2007;110(3):614–624.

9. Downard CD, Rapkin LB, Gow KW. Melanoma in children and adolescents. *Surg Oncol.* 2007;16(3):215–220.

10. Tannous ZS, Mihm MC Jr, Sober AJ, Duncan LM. Congenital melanocytic nevi: clinical and histopathologic features, risk of melanoma, and clinical management. *J Am Acad Dermatol*. 2005;52(2):197–203.

11. Zaal LH, Mooi WJ, Klip H, van der Horst CM. Risk of malignant transformation of congenital melanocytic nevi: a retrospective nationwide study from the Netherlands. *Plast Reconstr Surg*. 2005;116(7):1902–1909.

12. DeDavid M, Orlow SJ, Provost N, et al. A study of large congenital melanocytic nevi and associated malignant melanomas: review of cases in the New York University Registry and the world literature. *J Am Acad Dermatol*. 1997;36(3 Pt 1):409–416.

13. Ruiz-Maldonado R, Tamayo L, Laterza AM, Duran C. Giant pigmented nevi: clinical, histopathologic, and therapeutic considerations. *J Pediatr*. 1992;120(6):906–911.

14. Paradela S, Fonseca E, Prieto VG. Melanoma in children. *Arch Pathol Lab Med*. 2011;135(3):307–316.

14a. Lu C, Zhang J, Nagahawatte P, et al. The genomic landscape of childhood and adolescent melanoma. *J Invest Dermatol*. 2015;135(3):816–23.

15. Navid F. *Genetic Alterations in Childhood Melanoma*. ASCO Educational Handbook; 2012:589-92.

16. Berg P, Wennberg AM, Tuominen R, et al. Germline *CDKN2A* mutations are rare in child and adolescent cutaneous melanoma. *Melanoma Res*. 2004;14(4):251–255.

17. Bradford PT, Goldstein AM, Tamura D, et al. Cancer and neurologic degeneration in xeroderma pigmentosum: long term follow-up characterises the role of DNA repair. *J Med Genet*. 2011;48(3):168–176.

18. Barnhill RL. The Spitzoid lesion: rethinking Spitz tumors, atypical variants, 'Spitzoid melanoma' and risk assessment. *Mod Pathol*. 2006;19 (Suppl 2):S21–S33.

19. Reed D, Kudchadkar R, Zager JS, Sondak VK, Messina JL. Controversies in the evaluation and management of atypical melanocytic proliferations in children, adolescents, and young adults. *JNCCN*. 2013;11(6):679–686.

20. Aldrink JH, Selim MA, Diesen DL, et al. Pediatric melanoma: a single-institution experience of 150 patients. *J Pediatr Surg*. 2009;44(8):1514–1521.

21. Han D MS, Han G, Messina JL, Sondak VK, Zager JS. The unique clinical characteristics of melanoma diagnosed in children. *Ann Surg Oncol*. 2012;19(12):3888–3895.

22. Howman-Giles R, Shaw HM, Scolyer RA, et al. Sentinel lymph node biopsy in pediatric and adolescent cutaneous melanoma patients. *Ann Surg Oncol*. 2010;17(1):138–143.

23. Mu E, Lange JR, Strouse JJ. Comparison of the use and results of sentinel lymph node biopsy in children and young adults with melanoma. *Cancer*. 2012;118(10):2700–2707.

24. Roaten JB, Partrick DA, Pearlman N, Gonzalez RJ, Gonzalez R, McCarter MD. Sentinel lymph node biopsy for melanoma and other melanocytic tumors in adolescents. *J Pediatr Surg*. 2005;40(1):232–235.

25. Mills OL, Marzban S, Zager JS, Sondak VK, Messina JL. Sentinel node biopsy in atypical melanocytic neoplasms in childhood: a single institution experience in 24 patients. *J Cutan Pathol*. 2012;39(3):331–336.

26. Han D, Zager JS, Han G, et al. The unique clinical characteristics of melanoma diagnosed in children. *Ann Surg Oncol*. 2012;19(12):3888–3895.

27. Parida L, Morrisson GT, Shammas A, et al. Role of lymphoscintigraphy and sentinel lymph node biopsy in the management of pediatric melanoma and sarcoma. *Pediatr Surg Int.* 2012;28(6):571–578.

28. Dale Han LMT, Reed DR, Messina JL, Sondak VK. The prognostic significance of lymph node metastasis in pediatric melanoma and atypical melanocytic proliferations. *Expert Rev Dermatol.* 2013;8(2):103–106.

29. Pearce MS, Salotti JA, Little MP, et al. Radiation exposure from CT scans in childhood and subsequent risk of leukaemia and brain tumours: a retrospective cohort study. *Lancet.* 2012;380(9840):499–505.

30. Lange JR, Palis BE, Chang DC, Soong SJ, Balch CM. Melanoma in children and teenagers: an analysis of patients from the National Cancer Data Base. *J Clin Oncol.* 2007;25(11):1363–1368.

31. Strouse JJ, Fears TR, Tucker MA, Wayne AS. Pediatric melanoma: risk factor and survival analysis of the surveillance, epidemiology and end results database. *J Clin Oncol.* 2005;23(21):4735–4741.

32. Averbook BJ, Lee SJ, Delman KA, et al. Pediatric melanoma: analysis of an international registry. *Cancer.* 2013; 119(22):4012–4019.

33. Ferrari A, Bono A, Baldi M, et al. Does melanoma behave differently in younger children than in adults? A retrospective study of 33 cases of childhood melanoma from a single institution. *Pediatrics.* 2005;115(3):649–654.

34. Moore-Olufemi S, Herzog C, Warneke C, et al. Outcomes in pediatric melanoma: comparing prepubertal to adolescent pediatric patients. *Ann Surg.* 2011;253(6):1211–1215.

35. Paradela S, Fonseca E, Pita-Fernandez S, et al. Prognostic factors for melanoma in children and adolescents: a clinicopathologic, single-center study of 137 patients. *Cancer.* 2010;116(18):4334–4344.

36. Kirkwood JM, Strawderman MH, Ernstoff MS, Smith TJ, Borden EC, Blum RH. Interferon alfa-2b adjuvant therapy of high-risk resected cutaneous melanoma: the Eastern Cooperative Oncology Group Trial EST 1684. *J Clin Oncol.* 1996;14(1):7–17.

37. Shah NC, Gerstle JT, Stuart M, Winter C, Pappo A. Use of sentinel lymph node biopsy and high-dose interferon in pediatric patients with high-risk melanoma: the Hospital for Sick Children experience. *J Pediatr Hematol Oncol.* 2006;28(8):496–500.

38. Navid F, Furman WL, Fleming M, et al. The feasibility of adjuvant interferon alpha-2b in children with high-risk melanoma. *Cancer.* 2005;103(4):780–787.

39. Wang YS, Youngster S, Bausch J, Zhang R, McNemar C, Wyss DF. Identification of the major positional isomer of pegylated interferon alpha-2b. *Biochemistry.* 2000;39(35):10634–10640.

40. Glue P, Fang JW, Rouzier-Panis R, et al. Pegylated interferon-alpha2b: pharmacokinetics, pharmacodynamics, safety, and preliminary efficacy data. Hepatitis C Intervention Therapy Group. *Clin Pharmacol Ther.* 2000;68(5):556–567.

41. Krepler C, Certa U, Wacheck V, Jansen B, Wolff K, Pehamberger H. Pegylated and conventional interferon-alpha induce comparable transcriptional responses and inhibition of tumor growth in a human melanoma SCID mouse xenotransplantation model. *J Invest Dermatol.* 2004;123(4):664–669.

42. Lindsay KL, Trepo C, Heintges T, et al. A randomized, double-blind trial comparing pegylated interferon alfa-2b to interferon alfa-2b as initial treatment for chronic hepatitis C. *Hepatology.* 2001;34(2):395–403.

43. Talpaz M, O'Brien S, Rose E, et al. Phase 1 study of polyethylene gly-col formulation of interferon alpha-2B (Schering 54031) in Philadelphia chromosome-positive chronic myelogenous leukemia. *Blood*. 2001;98(6):1708–1713.

44. Eggermont AM, Suciu S, Santinami M, et al. Adjuvant therapy with pegylated interferon alfa-2b versus observation alone in resected stage III mela-noma: final results of EORTC 18991, a randomised phase III trial. *Lancet*. 2008;372(9633):117–126.

45. Eggermont AM, Suciu S, Testori A, et al. Ulceration and stage are predic-tive of interferon efficacy in melanoma: results of the phase III adjuvant trials EORTC 18952 and EORTC 18991. *Eur J Cancer*. 2012;48(2):218–225.

46. Bukowski RM, Tendler C, Cutler D, Rose E, Laughlin MM, Statkevich P. Treating cancer with PEG Intron: pharmacokinetic profile and dos-ing guidelines for an improved interferon-alpha-2b formulation. *Cancer*. 2002;95(2):389–396.

46a. Chapman PB, Hauschild A, Robert C, et al. Improved survival with vemurafenib in melanoma with BRAF V600E mutation. *N Engl J Med*. 2011;364(26):2507–2516.

46b. Hauschild A, Grob JJ, Demidov LV, et al. Dabrafenib in BRAF-mutated meta-static melanoma: a multicentre, open-label, phase 3 randomised controlled trial. *Lancet*. 2012;380(9839):358–365.

46c. Flaherty KT, Puzanov I, Kim KB, et al. Inhibition of mutated, activated BRAF in metastatic melanoma. *N Engl J Med*. 2010;363(9):809–819.

46d. Sosman JA, Kim KB, Schuchter L, et al. Survival in BRAF V600-mutant advanced melanoma treated with vemurafenib. *N Engl J Med*. 2012;366(8):707–714.

46e. Larkin J, Ascierto PA, Dreno B, et al. Combined vemurafenib and cobimetinib in BRAF-mutated melanoma. *N Engl J Med*. 2014;371(20): 1867–1876.

46f. Long GV, Stroyakovskiy D, Gogas H, et al. Combined BRAF and MEK inhibition versus BRAF inhibition alone in melanoma. *N Engl J Med*. 2014;371(20):1877–1888.

46g. Robert C, Karaszewska B, Schachter J, et al. Improved overall survival in melanoma with combined dabrafenib and trametinib. *N Engl J Med*. 2015;372(1):30–39.

46h. McArthur GA, Ribas A. Targeting oncogenic drivers and the immune system in melanoma. *J Clin Oncol*. 2013;31(4):499–506.

46i. Hodi FS, O'Day SJ, McDermott DF, et al. Improved survival with ipilimumab in patients with metastatic melanoma. *N Engl J Med*. 2010;363(8):711–723.

46j. Robert C, Thomas L, Bondarenko I, et al. Ipilimumab plus dacarba-zine for previously untreated metastatic melanoma. *N Engl J Med*. 2011;364(26):2517–2526.

46k. Schadendorf D, Hodi FS, Robert C, et al. Pooled analysis of long-term sur-vival data from phase II and phase III trials of ipilimumab in unresectable or metastatic melanoma. *J Clin Oncol*. 2015;33(17):1889–1894.

46l. Maio M, Grob JJ, Aamdal S, et al. Five-year survival rates for treatment-naive patients with advanced melanoma who received ipilimumab plus dacarbazine in a phase III trial. *J Clin Oncol*. 2015;33(10):1191–1196.

46m. Robert C, Long GV, Brady B, et al. Nivolimab in previously untreated mela-noma without BRAF mutation. *New Engl J Med*. 2015;372(4): 320–330.

46n. Weber JS, D'Angelo SP, Minor D, et al. Nivolumab versus chemotherapy in patients with advanced melanoma who progressed after anti-CTLA-4 treatment (CheckMate 037): a randomised, controlled, open-label, phase 3 trial. *Lancet Oncol.* 2015;16(4):375–384.

46o. Postow MA, Chesney J, Pavlick AC, et al. Nivolumab and ipilimumab versus ipilimumab in untreated melanoma. *N Engl J Med.* 2015;372(21):2006–2017.

46p. Robert C, Schachter J, Long GV, et al. Pembrolizumab versus ipilimumab in advanced melanoma. *N Engl J Med.* 2015;372(26):2521–2532.

46q. Eggermont AMM, Chiarion-Sileni V, Grob JJ, et al. Adjuvant ipilimumab versus placebo after complete resection of high-risk stage III melanoma (EORTC 18071): a randomised, double-blind, phase 3 trial. *Lancet Oncol.* 2015;16(5):522–530.

47. Schmid-Wendtner MH, Paerschke G, Baumert J, Plewig G, Volkenandt M. Value of ultrasonography compared with physical examination for the detection of locoregional metastases in patients with cutaneous melanoma. *Melanoma Res.* 2003;13(2):183–188.

48. Kaste SC, Pappo AS, Jenkins JJ 3rd, Pratt CB. Malignant melanoma in children: imaging spectrum. *Pediatr Radiol.* 1996;26(11):800–805.

48a. Sreeraman Kumar R, Messina JL, Sondak, VK, et al. Treating melanoma in adolescents and young adults: challenges and solutions. *Clin Oncol in Adole and Young Adults.* Accepted. September, 2015.

Index

Page numbers followed by *f* or *t* indicate figures or tables.

163